Curly

A Survivor's Story

...The Breast is Yet to Come...

Joan Fraser Yeash BSN, RN

Curly

A Survivor's Story

...The Breast is Yet to Come...

By Joan Fraser Yeash, BSN, RN

Forward by Dr James M Yeash

First Edition: November 2006

Published by lulu.com

ISBN: 978-0-6151-3693-6

Cover design and layout by James M Yeash

Dedication

To my wonderful, loving family: James, my better half and the love of my life, and my children, Jerred, Ryan, Justin, Erik, and Kate who never once thought that I would do anything but survive. They put up with a lot of tears and many late nights and early mornings.

To my sister, Janet, brother, Harvey and sister-in-law Kitty, and my niece, Heather, and Gerianne, for their sometimes agonizing help editing this book.

To my late mother, Jean, who taught me to love, and my father, Harvey, who taught me to fight, and to my mother-in-law, Kathryn Svistak Yeash, who thankfully gave birth to my husband, and accepted me into my extended family 25 years ago and has provided so much help and love to me and my family.

To my wonderful friends who I mention throughout the book for their prayers and support.

Many thanks to my health care team, the late Dr Jeff Clarke and Drs Rebecca Wiebe, Debora Ma, John Fleagle, and Fran Mason, who helped me survive, as well as JoAnn Henritze for helping me exercise through it all, and Rocky Mountain Team Survivor-Boulder, headed by Dora, my cancer surviving companions who believe exercising together through cancer is the best treatment. Thanks also to Keith Jaroslow for inspiration and editing.

And to God, who put these people in my life, and is my constant companion on the journey.

Contents

FORWARD

As a family physician for over twenty years, I have had the opportunity on many occasions to help patients and their families deal with a cancer diagnosis. Although any cancer diagnosis is devastating, breast cancer represents a personal attack on the outward appearance of a woman. It directly affects nearly one in seven women and indirectly millions more. It is a cancer that can be both disfiguring and fatal, and is a battle against a disease as well as the emotional and psychological effects that occur when a woman no longer feels whole.

For a period of several months, I supported and struggled with my own wife Joan's fight against breast cancer. I had my faith in medicine and medical technology shaken, and my faith in God tested. I tried to provide the physical and emotional support that was needed, the best that I could, as the love of my life was being brought to her lowest point. The woman who had always been a pillar of strength to me, and seemed to be strong in all the areas in which I had weaknesses, was slowly and completely humiliated.

The name of the book comes from what happened to Joan's hair as a result of chemotherapy. Curly also represents the twists and turns that life takes in what literally became a challenge to continue living. I had never seen Joan in such pain and anguish. I had never seen her fearful of what was to come. I had never seen her any other way than self-assured and strong.

We learned to appreciate each other more, as well as how fortunate we are to have such wonderful friends, family and neighbors. We learned that God is always with us even in the loneliest moments. This book represents a journey that we took reluctantly, but with determination, and the guarded belief that all of us would make it through successfully. I will never say that Joan's breast cancer was a good thing, but it did help us focus on what is really important, and spiritually reawaken us to the blessings of living and loving and caring that maybe we had taken for granted. This is a lot easier to see retrospectively.

'Curly' chronicles a year in the life of my wife Joan during her fight against breast cancer. It is a very personal and spiritual account from a nurse's perspective of what so many women go through with the hope that they too can ultimately and proudly be called survivors.

Jim Yeash

Part 1
Chapter 1
Family Background

Early in September 2002, before cancer became the center of my life, while working out on my elliptical trainer, I enjoyed some much needed time to myself. My five children returned to school. My children, Jerred (age 19) and the only one away from home in college, Ryan (age 16), Justin (age 15), Erik (age 12), and last but not least my only daughter, Kate (age 6). Kate was the joy of my life and kept me young. I felt as if I had emerged from a dark and winding tunnel. It had been an extremely stressful summer, but I felt a wonderful aura of freedom spread through me. It was a beautiful late summer day and my 47th birthday. That birthday was one to be remembered as it was the day I found a small lump in my left breast.

Except for childbirth, I had very little past medical history. I treated my body very well and exercised faithfully for over 20 years. I believed in preventative care, received physical examinations when I was supposed to and stayed current with age appropriate screening tests. My risk for any life-threatening disease was extremely low. Cancer was virtually nonexistent in my family except a first cousin diagnosed with breast cancer at the age of 36 and her brother with neck cancer. My mother and grandmother had both died of stroke related illnesses and I believed that I needed to take preventative measures against coronary heart disease. I ate a healthy diet and always tried to get enough sleep, but I led a very busy and high pressured life, which required significant time management and prioritization.

Four years ago, I had been diagnosed with Benign Paroxysmal Positional Vertigo (BPPV). I woke up in the middle of the night and the room was spinning. Making my way into the bathroom was impossible on two feet because I could not stand up because my world was literally out of control. I ended up crawling since I knew where the floor was. BPPV was related to tiny little particles in the inner ear. These little particles mobilized and floated around the inner ear causing extreme dizziness when my head position changed. I became so depressed at the time and the thought of living with the dizziness became horrifying. Within the next several weeks, I found out how very insignificant the dizziness was.

I was the youngest child of older parents. My mother at 35 years of age in 1955, the year I was born, was pretty old by the standards of the day. My sister Janet and brother Harvey preceded me by nine and twelve years respectively. I was almost a second family for my parents and we developed a unique bond. My brother and sister say I had a privileged upbringing. I was very disciplined, and as such was included in events that other children my age rarely if ever experienced. I dined at the finest restaurants and met many national and international dignitaries because I was well-mannered and a proper General's daughter. I had spoken to Dwight Eisenhower on the parade field at the United States Military Academy. Ambassadors graced our home in South Dakota. Astronaut and personal friend Col Frank Borman was a frequent visitor during the late 1960's. One of my father's prized possessions was a photo signed by him that was taken in December 1968. The photograph was of the earth as seen during the first orbit around the moon by a manned spacecraft.

My mother was an intelligent, graceful and lovely woman, and a very good role model for healthcare. She had been conscientious and wise before her time in taking care of herself. Perhaps the diagnosis of breast cancer in our neighbor and good friend in 1969 frightened her. She set an excellent example for me to follow. She was also a terrific role model as a physically active mother and devoted wife. Up until age 75, she was an avid golfer and tennis player. By 1996, her health had been deteriorating as a result of a potpourri of bizarre medical events and multiple small strokes over the preceding several years. My father had a difficult time believing that the 'setbacks' were anything other than transient. He believed that for every illness, there was a cure, and as the nurse, I should have figured this out and solved the problem. (Or so he kept telling me) Surely Jim, my physician husband would solve anything I couldn't. Even with the apparent erosion of her quality of life, she seemed very comfortable and happy. From the perspective of the rest of the family, especially my father, her quality of life was not optimal.

Activities that she enjoyed doing for years, like reading books, writing letters, and visiting with friends were no longer of interest to her. She answered questions, but rarely initiated conversation. She looked young and those who had not known her previously thought she was in good health.

In spite of this, she seemed quite content. I learned through this experience that sometimes you have to accept life as it is and make the most of it, and my mother seemed to be able to do that now.

In my early years, we lived in a picturesque, historic five bedroom house overlooking the lush, green Hudson River Valley. In retrospect, while growing up at West Point, I was exposed to a plethora of environmental toxins. There were times when each week during the summer we were exposed to pesticides that were sprayed from drive-by fogger trucks in hopes of controlling the mosquito population. After that, I also lived on a golf course for seven years where fertilizer and pesticides were frequently applied. I never really thought much about these environmental toxins until my life was jeopardized by a potentially fatal disease.

My father had smoked excessively when he was younger, and although he quit before I was born, his 86 years had begun to take their toll. This man had been the backbone of the family since he and my mother were married. He had severe degenerative arthritis and had several back surgeries and procedures that recently rendered him unable to continue his role as my mother's primary caretaker in the assisted care facility where they lived not far from my home.

In 1996, as my mother was becoming unable to compensate for a series of mini-strokes, it became clear to my dad that they should live near one of their children and move into an environment that was less independent. He asked me to find a suitable place for them near my community in the Boulder-Louisville area of Colorado. Not only was this a scenic and attractive area to live, but such a move would enable them to share in the lives of their five younger grandchildren and later their oldest granddaughter, Heather and her two girls, who were the first of the great grand-children. I looked forward to that. At this point, I became the primary family member caretaker. My daughter and fifth child Kate was born in August of 1996, so I cared for my young family and my aging parents as well.

This move added a new dimension to my life and to theirs. While they were not thrilled to have to depend on me, they were both in reasonably good health and relatively independent at that time, and I was certainly healthy enough to accept the challenge. Having them nearby was a wonderful experience for our family and we spent most holidays and special times together. However, as their health began to deteriorate and their demands increased, I began to feel the added stress.

For months, it seemed that I bounced back and forth between the assisted care facility, emergency rooms, hospitals, operating rooms, and the nursing home visiting my mother and father during their numerous stays at the various health care facilities. When I finally got my parents back together in the same room at the nursing home in July 2002, I was thrilled. The staff was very accommodating moving residents around so that my mom and dad could be roommates. At one point my father exhibited very bizarre behaviors explained away because he was heavily medicated for severe back pain and anxiety. My mother just contentedly shrugged her shoulders. I received numerous phone calls and had many expectations from my parents and from various nursing personnel at the different facilities. I began to feel increasingly more run down. I hadn't been eating and exercising as I should, and my family demands never went away, so at this point, I knew I was ready to implode.

I rationalized that my fatigue could easily be attributed to having so much going on in my life. I continued to make frequent hospital and nursing home visits to help my parents. My sister had been able to adjust her schedule and come to help out, as had my brother. I had scheduled a mammogram months before and it happened to fall during the period of time that my father was having one of his several hospitalizations in July 2002. I thought about canceling, but my sister Janet encouraged me to go ahead with the appointment. It was important for women to take care of themselves and follow the medical recommendations for breast cancer screening. I performed a self breast examination the day of my mammogram. Everything felt normal, no unusual lumps or bumps. As with most women, my anxiety always rose prior to having a mammogram. I had a suspicious reading in 1998 that required a shortened interval follow-up, which added to the stress that I did not need at this time. A week later a normal report arrived in the mail so I felt that I had nothing to worry about.

I hired extra caregivers to help take care of my parents with the hope of preventing injuries to either of them, as well as help with the little problems that arose from time to time. Skilled nursing facilities were notoriously frightening places for family members because most were extremely short staffed. Everyone always needed something immediately and therefore acted impetuously, which led to injuries for the patients. When many call bells were ringing, it was hard to know which to answer first. Before you knew it, something catastrophic happened.

My sister went home and I thought things were improving. My parents would be celebrating their 62nd anniversary on July 31st and I ordered a big cake to have at lunch in the nursing home dining facility. I found these retirement homes and communities disquieting because deaths were frequent among the population. On the first floor of the skilled nursing facility, there was a hospice care center that I passed by in order to get on the elevator to the skilled nursing area. While death seemingly surrounded me, it had little impact on me. I was always on a mission and tried not to dwell on it.

Having been on an emotional roller coaster for the entire summer, 2002 would not go down as one of our most stress-free. We did get a quick break in August and my family and I left for Vail, Colorado for a soccer tournament and a relaxing weekend in the mountains. I was still exhausted from the events of the summer and I let Justin, my fifteen year old son with his learner's permit, drive the car to the mountains. Letting a teenager drive my car in the mountains was probably not the best way to alleviate my already high level of stress, but somehow this seemed to be an escape from my usual stressors. When my husband arrived a few days into the tournament, instead of celebrating some family time, I had a nagging feeling that I should return home. I did not know why I was overcome by that feeling. Jim would be there with Justin, the soccer player, and therefore I should go home to check on the status of my parents. Jim quickly dissuaded me as this really was going to be the only time we would have to spend together as a family all summer. We always seemed to be too busy to really relax. With five children and a busy husband, we had to work hard to find time together.

Believe me, we chose to have five children and had no regrets, but with their wide range in ages, it was a challenge to get everyone together for a leisurely vacation. The next day was Sunday and the last day of the tournament, so I decided to stay. I saw two games and had a very unsettled feeling that I needed to get home right away. Justin had played his last game and the team placed, for them, a disappointing third place, but that still qualified them for a National Tournament in Orlando, Florida in January. I left immediately and the traffic on the trip home from Vail was very heavy, but not unusual for a Sunday afternoon return from the mountains. After running into a road closure and becoming temporarily lost, I was an hour late getting home leaving me no time to visit my folks at the nursing home, a decision I would later regret. Exhausted after a busy weekend, I fell into my own bed for a good night's sleep.

At ten fifteen, we were awakened by a call from the nurse at the skilled nursing facility. Exhausted, I cringed and looked at Jim and thought out loud, "Oh no what could possibly have happened?" Although it was not unusual to get late night calls, I knew that this had to be bad news. The nurse reported that my mother fell when she tried to get off the toilet without the aide's assistance. She told me that my mother was somewhat incoherent and fading in and out of consciousness. I tried to clear my thoughts. I knew her symptoms were serious and we needed to do something quickly. She was deteriorating rapidly neurologically. I requested that the ambulance take her to the hospital, where I would meet them in the Emergency Room. That was August 4th, 2002.Overcome by a sudden chill, I threw on clothes and a jacket. I left in haste, not knowing exactly what to expect. Arriving at the Emergency Department, I found my mother comatose and unresponsive.

On the morning of August 5th, my mother passed away. We had some sense of peace knowing she was comfortable and died quickly, peacefully, with dignity and with many of her loving family at her side.

Believing the decisions and stress associated with the death of a loved one to be behind me, it was now September and I tried to keep up my normal daily family routine. My children were very busy, for which I was pleased, but it took quite a bit of coordination on my part to get them everywhere they needed to be.

I was very tired but I attributed that to the series of stressful life events throughout the summer. I believed strongly in the stress theory of illness, so I knew I needed somehow to relax and get some meaningful and much needed rest and recuperation. I had always believed since college that stress negatively impacts health by decreasing the ability of the immune system to ward off illness. If the immune system is not functioning at capacity, opportunistic diseases can take hold and cause serious illness.

During my private time I exercised. I screamed or cried or talked to people who were not there and I talked and prayed to God. I had a lot of questions for Him. Still mourning my mother's death, I learned that my favorite chaplain from my youth had committed suicide. This man had been my most influential Christian figure growing up at the United States Military Academy. He was the Cadet Chaplain for a number of years and later went on to become the Chaplain of the US Senate. I was devastated by both the news of his death and the means by which he died. He and his family were in my prayers that day. Death seemed to be stalking those I cared about. I was troubled and I prayed harder. Sometimes my prayer was a running dialog. My children have asked with whom I was speaking. My lips must move and on occasion I suppose that I spoke out loud. Sometimes I talked to myself and sometimes to God. As a mother of five who also took care of an aging parent, I had earned the right to talk to myself.

It was the ninth of September, and for someone on her 47th birthday I felt good about myself after an hour of aerobic workout and a bit of weight training. I got into the shower to clean up and realized that it had been two months since I had done a self breast exam.

I hadn't been overly concerned since I had the normal mammogram report in July. The summer had been quite tumultuous and I thought to myself that this was the perfect time to get back a little normalcy in my life. As I checked the left breast and then the right, something was wrong. I checked the left side again. I was sure I felt a lump the size of a small pea in the upper, outer part of my left breast. I tried to rationalize it away. How could this be? I had a normal mammogram just six weeks before and I had not felt the lump then. Unfortunately, on that day, my birthday, the lump was most certainly there. I was sure it was cancer and that explained my fatigue. As a woman and a nurse, over time I had learned to listen to my intuition. I spent years in the Intensive Care Unit and Emergency Department. I sensed when a patient was about to have a cardiac arrest and when it would be a particularly difficult shift. I learned to trust my intuition because more often than not it was eerily accurate. Unfortunately, my intuition would prove to be correct once again.

Chapter 2

Happy Birthday and the First Diagnosis

So Happy Birthday to me. I had a lump in my breast. Even my husband Jim, always the calm one who understates everything, agreed that it should be removed. I was stunned because he never reacted so quickly to anything health related in the family. I knew I was in trouble, but it was small and I had just found it. I thought that would be to my advantage. Jim found out at about the same time, that one of his uncles for whom he was named, had died so he left suddenly to return to Pennsylvania for the funeral. The timing was not great but then we really had no control. Could anything more, possibly happen? I kicked myself after saying that because there was always something more that could happen. I tried to gather my wits and made a plan. Plans were good. Great Armies had plans, so I should too. Nurses were always making Care Plans; now the only difference was I was my own patient and planned my own care I called a surgeon and made an appointment after Jim told me of a general surgeon in Wheat Ridge that his patients and several nurses liked and respected. In my mind, nurses were the greatest gauge. They were very critical. The surgeon I had always been sure would be there for the family had retired two years earlier. I wanted to bring him out of retirement.

Getting through to the surgeon's office was easy but I could not be seen until September 24th. I wanted to be seen immediately. I could wait or maybe not. I certainly did not want to create chaos by telling them I wanted an appointment right away even if it was for my peace of mind. Then I called for an appointment with my family physician. He had an opening on the 18th. He could have seen me a bit sooner but I would have missed one of the children's games. It was only nine days. I told no one what was happening and just ruminated quietly about it. I thought I was in control. I checked the lump at least 100 times a day to make sure it was still there.

A little obsession was good. It kept me on my toes. I finally saw my doctor. He was not overly concerned and thought we could watch it for a month to see what one menstrual cycle did to the lump. Sometimes these lumps just disappeared. I was not really excited with that so he suggested an ultrasound and I told him I already had an appointment with a surgeon because I was just not comfortable waiting. His suggestion remained, to get the ultrasound. The ultrasound machine malfunctioned when the technician tried to send pictures to the radiologist. Nothing surprised me anymore, since I was convinced that if anything could go wrong it would, particularly when it came to a health care practitioner's healthcare. The radiologist finally received the pictures and also thought the breast looked normal. I should have felt relieved. After all, within a span of two months I had a normal mammogram and normal ultrasound. Although some people thought I was making a mountain out of an ant hill, I was still going to see the surgeon. And regardless of the potential effects that the monthly cycling of estrogen and progesterone might have on the lump, I was just not comfortable waiting.

On the 24th I drove alone to see the surgeon with my normal mammogram and normal ultrasound in hand. My appointment had been scheduled at four in the afternoon. Why in the world did anyone go anywhere during rush hour? I thought again to myself that I must be over-reacting and there was really nothing there in my breast. My denial kicked in and I knew it. The surgeon's office was foreboding when I walked in. There was cancer information everywhere and a TLC catalog which had wigs and hats for hair loss during chemotherapy. I remembered looking at the catalog thinking those women looked pretty in hats and wigs. I could be a hat person even though they gave me a headache. In blissful ignorance I thought, I won't need any hats. I finally saw the surgeon and I liked her a lot. She seemed very empathetic and personable. She asked me to find the lump for her since she hadn't even felt it at first, then she palpated again and agreed it was the size of a tiny pea. It really was there after all and my heart sank. Up until this point, I hoped that I had overreacted. Actually, I kept hoping that the lump wasn't really there. I then had to make my first decision. Did I want to have a needle biopsy or excision biopsy done? She told me, also, that the lump was probably benign and it was very small. There was only a 10 percent chance that the lump was malignant, but, I wanted it out. I could have had a needle aspiration that day in the office and known the results right away, but there was a possibility that she could miss the mass in my breast with the needle and I was not willing to risk that. I opted to have an excision biopsy that could take several days to schedule. By this time my lump might as well have been the size of a grapefruit. I think any normal person would have gone with the immediate gratification of the needle biopsy but the health care provider side wanted to be absolutely sure. She and I scheduled the excision biopsy for two days later at the hospital located five minutes from my home. It seemed as if I were watching myself in a movie. It was so surreal and yet I was captivated. Two agonizing days later seemed like an eternity. Of course changing schedules around was tough but Jim and I both managed to get our affairs in order. Rearranging the lives for a family of seven was quite a logistical feat. At this point I finally shared the news with my good friends Nancy and Geri who both covered their worry as I confidently told them that the chances were good that the lump was actually nothing. They tentatively accepted this explanation. Geri and I had been friends since Junior High and I thought perhaps she sensed my anxiety. I pretended that everything was fine hoping no one saw through to my burgeoning fear.

The day came for the biopsy and I was allowed no food or water after midnight. That was NPO in nursing lingo. Light-headed, nauseous and very irritable because my stomach churned with hunger, I counted the minutes until I could leave for the hospital and get some sedation, since I wanted to relax, at least briefly. I did not want to be too sedated, though, because I wanted to ask questions and see the biopsy. I wanted to make sure that no one made a mistake. I actually drove myself to the hospital since Jim worked half a day. After all this was *just* a hoop I had to jump through.

The woman in the preoperative area, not far from me, was having a breast lump excision, better known as a lumpectomy and lymph nodes removed for biopsy. She, of course, knew already that she had breast cancer. She was in tears. Thank God, that was not me!

I was in and out of the operating room in 45 minutes. It was a very scary place, even to me and I had spent a lot of time in the Operating Room as a nurse or a student. I could only imagine how frightening it was for someone not familiar with a hospital. When you were being wheeled around on the bed you were totally vulnerable. I lost control of everything that was routine in my life and was totally at the mercy of these people, who did not even know me. The room was really cold and I felt a bit groggy but I was still asking questions. What was everyone doing? What anesthesia did I get? Which operating room was I in? I decided the medicine made me pretty chatty and maybe they wished I were a little less so. I felt a little prick as the lidocaine (numbing medicine) was injected into my breast and then I only felt pressure. It was nice to be awake and not feel anything. I felt and heard a pop when the surgeon removed the lump. I asked what it looked like. Of course, I wanted to see this lump before they sent it away and the surgeon showed it to me. The surgeon and pathologist both thought the lump looked benign. I felt a little silly making such a big deal out of this. Here I had been in the operating room and recovery room taking space away from a real sick person. However, I had a sinking feeling that all was not right. I could not put my finger on anything specific. The biopsy would normally be back in 48 hours but this was a Thursday, so it would be Monday the 30th before I got the results. I waited an extra day. Ignorance was truly bliss. At last I had a restful weekend. Not knowing anything was not a bad feeling.

Monday rolled around and, as always, was chaotic. I was anxious all day, since I knew I would receive the results. I kept my cell phone on and with me the whole day. I took Kate to dance class at 3:30 and returned home to get Justin and Erik both to different places at the same time. One went to soccer and the other to football. I thought it might be too late for any doctor to call results back to me.

I had just about given up for the day, when the phone rang at 4:30 and my heart almost stopped. It was my surgeon. She said, "Joan, I just can't believe this, I don't have good news. I never suspected this but your lump was cancerous."

Cancer, the big C. I was quiet initially and then started to ask questions. I wanted to see the pathology report. She faxed it to me. The doctor said she wanted to see me the next day as soon as my husband and I could get there. I decided on 5:00 pm since Jim had a full work day and this was the least disruptive time to schedule an appointment. The doctor asked if she should call Jim. At first I said no and then quickly said yes because he had many questions too, and I was not up to answering them. I wrote down everything as she told me all the information. I was able to maintain a clinical, non emotional level of functioning although I felt as if I were crawling out of my own skin. As an ex-military nurse, I could always count on my ability to be very clinical to get me through difficult times when I was working, like deaths, codes, car accidents, and ambulance runs. I had an uncanny ability to separate myself from a situation and remain a third party observer almost as if I played a movie role. After I got off the phone, none of the notes I had taken made any sense, so clearly I was not functioning at full capacity.

The surgeon gave me a lot of information in rapid succession. At one point I was sure I could not comprehend any more but it just kept coming. I needed to find a plastic surgeon and a medical oncologist. I should talk to several before I decided on any one. I also needed to talk to a radiation oncologist. She also told me to look over Dr. Susan Love's Breast Cancer book. It was full of information but the surgeon wanted to know what I thought of it from a nurse's perspective going through cancer, so she would know if it was a good resource to recommend. With the appointment set up, I got off the phone. I quickly reached information overload and was sure that my head would explode.

Two of my kids had heard the conversation and already knew the results were not good. I talked to them and reassured them and dropped them off at their respective destinations. I then had to pick Kate up at dance class. She was signed up to be on the dance competition team for the next year. I was beginning to reconsider how smart that commitment had been, but all I thought of now was keeping the disruption in our lives as minimal as possible. I hadn't cried yet and managed to get into the studio and told the dance teacher that I had just gotten the results of a biopsy and I had breast cancer. Then the flood gates opened. The words spilled out of my mouth for the first time. "I just found out that I have breast cancer."   I told her it would impact a lot, in the next few months, but I just could not talk about it until I knew more.

I burst into tears and she gave me a hug and I left before many people saw me crying. I just could not bear to tell anyone this news. It was almost as if I was ashamed of it. How could you be ashamed of having cancer? I hadn't done anything to be ashamed of. I hadn't chosen this to happen and I certainly had no control over it either. But, I felt damaged and almost dirty. I felt a new compassion for the lepers in the Bible. I tried to keep some composure as my six year old daughter and I talked on the way home. Yes, I was alright, but I needed to do more because the lump they took out was not a good one. I could not hold back the tears. "Mommy, why are you crying if it's going to be alright?" Kate asked. Good question. As I walked in the door of my house, the phone rang and it was Jim wondering how I was, but he needed to pick up one of the kids and go to another's game so I couldn't reflect on my feelings. I sobbed when I got off the phone. What should I do and who should be told? I called my dad and told him I had breast cancer but could not talk right now. Mom had just died. How could I possibly manage without my mom and best friend? How could my family go through any more? I called my sister who was always very thoughtful and she told me how good it was that I found the cancer when I did. It was very small and it might be gone completely. She had always been good at making me feel better. I did not feel better, though. I couldn't call my brother so my sister called him for me. My family doesn't cry and I did not want him to hear my voice cracking. We were a military family and we've been through wars. We don't cry or show emotion. We took care of business and moved on. Of course within minutes my brother called and wanted details or as many as I had. I got through the list for him in tears. I then called my friend Geri in Ft Collins, Colorado and she was stunned. She just could hardly speak and there was nothing either of us could say anyway. That was what was nice about good friends. Messages were conferred without talking. I went across the street to see my friend Nancy. She answered the door and I burst into tears. She just gave me a hug, since I did not even have to tell her the results because she just knew. What could anyone say? I knew everyone wanted to know what was next but I was not prepared to talk about it. Everyone wanted to be comforting but just didn't know quite how.

Jim finally got home about eight that night. I had no idea how either game turned out. I forgot to ask. I was just so glad to get him home. We talked and got the kids to bed or at least to their rooms so we could discuss my diagnosis in more detail. Jim thought he should be the one to get cancer not me. He said I had always done everything right. I exercised regularly, I ate a healthy diet, I saw the doctor when I should, and I didn't smoke. My risk for breast cancer should have been minimal. Yet here I was with a breast cancer diagnosis. My one risk for breast cancer was being a woman. One doesn't need any more risk than that. We both just could not imagine how this happened. A few weeks ago we mourned the loss of my mother and now we felt like we had been hit by a truck. We slept poorly that night. I cried every time I awakened because I was angry to find out that this was not just a bad dream. This was the beginning of many months of sleepless nights.

Medical science had totally let me down like a sinking lifeboat. I started getting mammograms at 35 years old, so I would have a baseline, from which all other mammograms could be compared and always felt very good when the results came back negative. I had ultrasounds during my pregnancies and they had always been accurate. The doctors were even able to tell the sex of each of the kids. Ultrasound had never let me down either although the results of one had been devastating. That had been the ultrasound confirming a diagnosis of anencephaly when I was six months pregnant with our second child. My second child, a daughter, named Mary had been found to have no cerebrum when I was 28 weeks pregnant. Basically, she had no brain, and therefore no brain function. She would not survive long after birth. The diagnosis had devastated the family. I could not begin to explain the utter hopelessness that followed this time in our lives. How could I ever receive another normal result and believe it? We believed Mary had been perfect. We had all come to rely on medical technology and I for one never believed it to be fallible. My entire career was spent doing tests on people and then getting the results. An action would follow that result. How many mistakes could have been made? On a more personal level, how many of my mammograms could have been read as normal, but were abnormal? How much earlier could this lump have been found and how much would my life be shortened because of this imperfect technology? I had gotten an abnormal result on a mammogram a few years ago on my left breast. I had a repeat mammogram done on that side and it was read as normal. Now I wondered, maybe I should have pursued that result. The blind trust of that follow up may haunt me for years.

How many other people had trusted technology and then died? In my thoughts these events snowballed out of control. The next day I needed to start calling doctors. How could God have done this to me? Hadn't I been through enough this year? As I tried to drift into sleep, my mind was filled with questions.

A few weeks earlier I had been talking with two of my 12 year old son's football coaches. A classmate of theirs had just gone through many episodes of chemotherapy and still died of breast cancer. They both agreed that if it had been them they would not have chosen the chemotherapy and would have chosen to die. I hesitated a moment and said I would go through chemotherapy if I knew that I would be cured. I knew that conversation would come back to me, I just didn't know how soon.

My children had very little reaction to my diagnosis of breast cancer. We did not tell my son in college for awhile and the others tried to be strong for my sake. They believed Jim from the beginning when he told them that the tumor was small and removed. He felt the diagnosis was blown out of proportion and most importantly, mom would be fine. I questioned them and not one child believed anything other than I would get better and cancer would not kill me.

Morning followed night, no matter how endless it seemed, and the alarm rang and another day began with my large family. There was no time to think and my appointment with the surgeon wasn't until five o'clock anyway. In the meantime, I ordered the book about breast cancer from the internet. I would not go into the bookstore to find it. Someone might think I had cancer. I did not want to admit that this was happening to me. I cried all the time when I was alone at home. I had to take my father to get an ingrown toenail removed at 2:00 pm so that took up some time. His primary care doctor was also mine. That was true Family Practice. I took a copy of the pathology report to put in my records and let him and his nurses know what was happening. Over the years the staff had become like family. They were there through the pregnancy with Kate at my age of 40. They had been through a lot of anxiety and a previous breast lump with me that indeed had gone away. One of the nurses came to mom's memorial service which had been very thoughtful. My family physician too was stunned and felt so badly for me. When we left he wished me good luck and told me to be in contact if I needed anything. That was the last time I saw him. Shortly after that visit, at the age of 46, he died from a heart attack while on a trail run. Was there no mercy? I found out he had taken my pathology report into his office, gotten my chart, looked over everything and cradled his shaking head in his hands. According to his two nurses, he tried to figure out if there was anything that he could have done differently that would have given him some idea of my diagnosis. Here again was another instance where someone had done everything right and the consequences were still tragic.

I tried to go on, I was a nurse and I knew the statistics. As I reminisced, I thought about my rotation through Pediatric Oncology at Walter Reed Army Medical Center. Those children had been so brave during their chemotherapy and many died. I could die from this. There was a huge weight on my shoulders. It felt like a truck being hauled around. I don't want radiation or chemotherapy. I just wanted this to be a horrible nightmare and to wake up. What did I do to deserve this? What had I done in my life to be dealt such a tragic hand? First I lost my mother, and prior to that my daughter Mary, and now I had to deal with breast cancer without either of them. I knew that God would not abandon me, but would carry me through the difficult times holding my hand the whole way. Yet, I still felt my faith being tested somehow. Memories of losing Mary our second child with anencephaly came flooding back. I remembered how empty I felt for months. I suddenly had that same awful gnawing feeling again. I wasn't sure we had seen God's hand in losing Mary yet. I arrived home just in time for Jim to pick me up and drive to Wheat Ridge to the appointment that I dreaded.

I felt dazed, going through the motions but not really aware of what I was doing. I put on my Fraser stoic face and braced myself trying to keep my mind clear so I could ask the hard questions. I felt like a freak. I did not want to cry in front of anyone. I had to be brave because that was how I was raised. I imagined unrealistically or not, that I had a blinking neon sign on my forehead that read *I have breast cancer*. When we entered the office there were pictures of breasts everywhere, sculptures and artwork. I don't remember seeing so many before. They seemed to come to life and as I picked them up they almost burned my hands. All the same catalogs and pamphlets were there but this time I took them with me. They were all about cancer and support groups and hats and wigs and breasts. I was getting really sick of breasts. The medical assistant put us in a room and gave me a copy of the book I had ordered earlier by Susan Love, so I looked at it. It was huge and felt like it weighed a ton sitting on my lap, not unlike the burden I felt I was carrying. The doctor came in and told us many of the same things she and I had discussed on the phone. The difference was Jim was with me hearing them, too, this time. Two sets of ears were better than one in this situation. Every now and then I got so overloaded that I couldn't listen to one more word. This was not the nurse in me whose quest was continually for more knowledge. This was the frightened woman. Intellectually, I understood everything that we were told, but emotionally I was incapable of processing all of the information. We went through options of care. Did I want a lumpectomy, a single mastectomy, or a double mastectomy? Would I like to have reconstruction right away and did I want implants or just muscle or both used in the reconstruction. If they used muscle only, it came from the abdomen, so I got a tummy tuck at the same time or they used a muscle from the back called the latisimus dorsi, but with that they use an implant too. That was far too much information to assimilate. I thought that a tummy tuck would be nice except that years later they found that many people got abdominal pain and hernias from the lack of support from the missing muscle and ended up in a girdle to support the abdominal organs. That was of course assuming they lived that long. So that didn't sound so good after all. The implants alone with out any muscle took several months to inflate and then lead to another surgery for placement of permanent ones. I saw my chest blown up with balloons. Over inflated and boom! I was just about to burst, just as I saw the implants. I was angry and afraid. The surgeon gave us the names of plastic surgeons, oncologists, and radiation oncologists, all of whom I was supposed to see. I needed to decide what I wanted to do and let her know. How could I do all this and maintain my schedule with my children? When I found the lump I had already planned a course of action, or at least I thought I had. No one knew this of course because I kept it to myself. I calmly told the surgeon that I would like a bilateral mastectomy, period. I don't need any reconstruction. I was not well endowed to begin with and this would not be an obvious change. Jim suggested that I might want to think about that decision. Typical male reaction, I thought! I agreed hesitantly. I had so many people to contact and appointments to be made. Right now the army health care system looked pretty good. It was the closest thing to socialized medicine that existed. They took care of everything and told you when to show up, sometimes all your appointments were within the same facility. This was a lot of work to accomplish for someone who cried every time she opened her mouth.

I really had to be proactive and get a grip on this. I was so overwhelmed that I could not even be rational.

I started to read about breast cancer that night and I tried to begin to formulate a plan. Assess, plan, implement, evaluate. I would never forget that being drilled into my head as a first year nursing student. The actual diagnosis I had was **ductal carcinoma, infiltrating, 8mm greatest diameter, moderately well differentiated extending to margin of biopsy**. It sounded like a death sentence to me, the woman, but to me, the nurse, it was not hopeless.

The nurse and the woman just cannot seem to get together on our thought processes. I still felt like medical science had let me down. About the same time an article came out in the news about Chinese women performing breast self-exams. The researchers found they were not very likely to find a lump, therefore, as a result of this study; we should rethink breast self-exams. I was livid. Medical science had let me down but I hadn't. Who knew when I might have found the tumor if ever, had I not faithfully performed breast self-exams monthly? At that moment I decided I would be a one woman force to teach anyone who would listen to not give up on breast self-exams because they were worthwhile and could find tumors early and could help save lives. I certainly hoped so, anyway. Also women needed to continue yearly mammograms after age forty but not use the results in isolation. An annual visit for a well woman exam was also still necessary with a thorough breast exam.

We were just about home and I needed to take Kate to soccer practice. My friend and neighbor Nancy brought dinner over and that was a blessing because food was the last thing I thought about at that time. My neighbors were exceedingly thoughtful. They were always there to help. It was hard for me to quit reading and researching all the information about breast cancer. Many things needed to be accomplished but I was obsessed with getting as much information as I could. I tried to read a few books and check the Internet for current information. It was October and Breast Cancer Awareness Month so there was no lack of information. How ironic! I could not get away from it. I really just wanted to know that I was normal in my reactions to everything that was going on because I felt my emotions were spiraling out of control. This long and agonizing day was finally over. Tomorrow I had many more tasks to accomplish.

Chapter 3

Doctors, doctors, doctors

The biopsy results were given to me on September 30th and the appointment with the General Surgeon took place the next day. On October 2nd I started calling plastic surgeons. I needed to find someone who could see me fairly soon. I called one doctor and made an appointment and then I called another whose office was closer. He was not actually taking new patients, but his office informed me that there was a new surgeon who had just started in my area. The office manager talked to the insurance company but the new surgeon was not yet on the plan. I was unhappy, but what could I do? The office manager talked to the original doctor and he agreed to see me because he knew Jim. I could see him that afternoon. Again Jim had to rearrange his schedule to accompany me to the appointment. Concentrating on seeing his patients was difficult at that time. I had previously scheduled myself to volunteer in Kate's class, so I decided to tell the guidance counselor at the school which two of my kids attended what had been happening since I really did not know how this ordeal was going to affect the children. If the kids started to do poorly in class or acted out I wanted the school to be understanding. I cried again when I told Kate's teacher what was going on with my health. Although being on the verge of tears, I managed to get through the time and functioned at least at a kindergarten level. I was able to say cancer out loud but I broke into tears whenever I did. It didn't get better the more times I said it. How would my children manage without me? How would my dad manage without me? I took care of his finances, ordered his medications, and dealt with all his health insurance issues. He was alone for the first time in 62 years. What would happen if I suddenly wasn't here? The answer to that question was just too much for me to handle at that time. I loved my family and didn't want to leave them prematurely but it was a possibility that I needed to deal with eventually.

I left school and walked to the plastic surgeon's office, which was close. I certainly was not fit to drive. Breast cancer patients needed to have a general surgeon to perform the mastectomy and a plastic surgeon to perform the reconstructive surgery. I really thought this whole health insurance thing was a pain. Surely socialized medicine must be better, but then on the *inside*, in the midst of chaos, the *outside* always seemed so much better. Those were my thoughts as I walked in the door at the office and met Jim. The office was serene with a waterfall in the corner and beautiful artwork, still too many pictures of women's breasts, but this was a plastic surgeon's office. What had I expected? The staff greeted us and as we walked in the phone rang. My insurance company was on the phone and had just given approval to the new female plastic surgeon and coverage would be effective on the 18th of the month, 16 days away. Would I like to see her instead today? She had time right away. I was thrilled. Of course I wanted to see her. There was something comforting about discussing this surgery with a woman. I made sure that her male counterpart was agreeable with my choice. I certainly didn't want to offend anyone. Twenty five years had hardened me a bit to male surgeons. I spent many hours in the operating room with them and I knew what they talked about. Nothing gave them more pleasure than embarrassing a young, naïve nursing student. We sat down in the office and waited for the doctor. I never thought I was very observant of my surroundings, but this office was beautiful. It was tastefully decorated and not typical of a doctor's office. It was so peaceful. The desk was huge and uncluttered. It turned out it was the other doctor's office, and when my doctor came in she informed us that her office was still full of boxes that had not been unpacked. So maybe he was a pretty good guy but I still wanted to see the female surgeon. We told each other our life stories. She had done her residency at Yale University and a fellowship in hand microsurgery in Los Angeles but she had done a lot of work with breast reconstruction and was very confident in her ability. She took out samples of the implants to show us. These days we had to use saline filled implants instead of silicone gel implants. I really preferred the feel of the gel better. She was going to try to get the silicone gel implants into a study here, but it would not be by the time I needed them.

I really started to like this doctor. She was personable and honest but she had no track record and all of the information I read suggested that I ask to see pictures. She had none, but showed me the work of the doctor with whom she shared the office. Somehow that just didn't bother me. She did an exam and got a really good look at my naked torso. Modesty had gone out the window by that time after baring my chest for doctors, nurses, and other health personnel. She talked about how my natural breasts draped. Yes, breasts drape. I learned so much. We then discussed the options available to me. I could get a bilateral mastectomy, removal of all of both breasts, which was already a given, and have implants put in that needed to be inflated at set periods of time until the skin was stretched enough for the real implant to be placed or I could have a procedure done in which she brought the latissimus dorsi muscle around from my back to cover an implant and when I woke up from surgery my breasts were there. Nothing had to be inflated. I asked about the abdominus rectus muscle procedure or TRAM flap, but she would not even consider doing this on me. It caused too many problems when both sides of the muscle had to be used when both breasts were reconstructed. She told me that I didn't have enough abdominal fat to even think about that procedure anyway. She really grew on me from that point forward.

Tentatively, I decided on the implant alone even though it tended to look like someone just plopped it on your chest but I agreed to do a bit more research and soul searching before I gave her my final decision. Having implants alone cut down the time I would have to be under anesthesia and in surgery. Not to mention recovery was much shorter. She had just started to build a private practice and I'm not even sure she was paid for our visit.

She was so frustrated with how slow the insurance companies were getting her credentialed that she was just seeing patients at no cost to build her practice. I asked if she could make my breasts larger than they were originally without it looking like too much. I had heard that male plastic surgeons had you coming out of surgery much larger than you thought. I apologize to all male plastic surgeons right now. The fact is you don't have breasts of any consequence and you don't have a clue. However I was not well endowed and as long as she was doing work, could I look better? The answer was a resolute, *absolutely*. When life gave you lemons, you made lemonade. I believed I might still have my sense of humor. She asked how big I was at the moment and where I wanted to be after surgery. I was currently an A cup and I'd like to be a B. That was not a problem. She just couldn't make me a D because again, I just didn't have enough fat or skin on my body for that. I really wanted to take fat from my behind and use it to make breasts. That wasn't a good idea, although there were a few places where that surgery was performed. Things started to look up just the slightest bit. Surgery still needed to be scheduled and she couldn't do it until after she took her plastic surgery boards. That was still fine with me. After an incredible three hour appointment with her we finally left with all our questions answered. I told her and the staff if they were looking for a nurse to employ to please let me know. I contemplated going back to work and I loved their office. I really had decided to go back to work, after eight years out of the work force, but, it looked more and more like that was not going to happen, at least not at that point in time.

The plastic surgery boards were on the 21st so I scheduled surgery after that day. I was certain that the cancer was metastasizing as each day dragged on. That was the woman again because the nurse knew that the tumor had probably taken 8 to 10 years to get to the point that I could feel it and now when I felt for it, it was gone. Waiting another week or two wouldn't affect the outcome of the surgery.

My husband Jim told his mother about the cancer and she was very upset, but offered to come out for a few weeks during the surgery. She had taken care of a family of five children and two mentally challenged brothers for her entire life. She had also taken care of my father-in-law who died of prostate cancer in 2001. She was as close to a saint as I would ever come. I was thankful for her offer because I worried about the kids maintaining some normalcy. They had to go to school and continue with their activities. This disease disrupted the family enough already. Even without a surgery date I started to look at how I would get everyone through this devastating ordeal.

More tumor markers came back. Tumor markers helped the oncologist to determine the best treatment. My tumor was estrogen and progesterone receptor positive but the Her2neu receptor was still questionable and more tests were needed. No big surprise there. If anything could go wrong or take longer, it seemed as if it would. This seemed to be the case with health care providers and their families. It looked negative which was a positive prognostic sign. In 20-25 percent of breast cancers, protein or genetic material was produced by the cancer cell. This could be measured and then the doctors could determine whether a woman was Her2neu positive or negative. The presence of this genetic material or oncogene might indicate a more aggressive tumor, but also could be treated with a drug called Herceptin. Herceptin involved weekly injections for a year. I was indeed Her2neu negative which was a small victory for me.

My primary surgeon left for a conference in San Francisco and nothing would happen without her. I did however get a surgery date scheduled. It was the 24th of October and I made all the preoperative appointments. The end was in sight or maybe it was just the beginning. I'm not quite sure which it was. Now I had to find a medical oncologist. I got a few names from Jim, my surgeon and friends and a couple were duplicates of other recommendations. I picked one after talking to the nursing staff and going online to read the biographies of everyone at the Rocky Mountain Cancer Center in Boulder. After playing a lot of phone tag I reached the scheduler and set up the appointment.

I actually said that I had just been diagnosed with breast cancer. I managed to get through the conversation without bursting into tears. I again felt as though I was watching myself in a movie. It did not seem real. As soon as I hung up the phone I burst into tears.

My sister, Janet, who was also a nurse, came to spend some time with our father and would accompany me to the oncology consultation. I was relieved because she was always so helpful when decisions had to be made. I thought it must come from experience. She would be my second set of ears and think of all the questions that I forgot. I still was not sleeping very well but I at least rested my poor battered body and had a lot of time to think. I prayed for a good outcome and I was still optimistic that no more cancer would be found.

In the meantime, my neighbors had slowly begun to learn of my diagnosis. It was so hard to tell people and as they learned of the news, they needed support from each other. This was my diagnosis but my friends were understandably frightened for me and for themselves and the vulnerability they all felt. When faced with this situation, it was really hard to know exactly what to do. My neighbor Lisa decided to put a box outside my door for people to drop by words of encouragement without having to ring the doorbell and disturb me. I did not want to face anyone. This was a lovely idea and indeed the notes from well wishers were plentiful. She dropped off a beautiful flowered box full of potpourri and it was already filled with encouraging Bible verses. As the days went by, more Bible verses were dropped off and cards and flowers. It was such a thoughtful gesture and reading all the uplifting notes made me cry. I knew people cared about me even if I was not able to talk to them about my cancer. I started to put those little Bible verses all over the house. I read them over and over again and even memorized some. Friends had lovingly picked out cards and words of inspiration that were very comforting.

In my mind I kept singing the old hymn, *O God Our Help in Ages Past*. I had always found the hymn particularly comforting. I preferred the old version, not the newly worded one. 'O God our help in ages past, our hope for years to come, our shelter from the stormy blast and our eternal home.' My childhood was spent at the United States Military Academy where my father was a permanent professor. Church was held in the exquisite Cadet Chapel with the most awe-inspiring organ I had ever heard. I found tremendous peace in going back to those childhood years and remembering the music.

All the old hymns and anthems that the cadet choir used to sing brought me such a sense of peace. Even though the peace was fleeting, it felt wonderful.

I was fraught with doubt the night before the appointment with the oncologist. I was afraid that I could not have the reconstruction because I might need chemotherapy or worse, radiation. Chemotherapy was very frightening to me because the side effects are so debilitating. I did not want chemo brain, heart failure, hair loss, or fatigue. I certainly did not want to spend the next months too sick to function. I had a lock on tired already. I knew radiation would have an absolutely devastating effect on breast implants so I tried not to even consider that option. It really was no wonder that I could not sleep at night. My brain never turned off.

The day arrived for the consult with the oncologist. Just saying that word was frightening. I searched hard to find him and had gotten recommendations from many sources, so I was pretty sure I would be happy with my choice. Truthfully, you should interview several before making a decision. My sister and I checked in and sat down to fill out the immense amount of paperwork. We were called fairly quickly, thankfully, because I found looking around at all the people in the waiting room distressing. Some wore hats, some were bald, some looked very sick. I wanted to jump up and say "I'm just here for a consultation! I don't really belong here. I am not sick." On our way back the medical assistant had me stand on the scale for a weight. She said every time I came in they would check my weight. What did she mean every time? I had no intention of needing to come back! I only had a small tumor and it had been removed. No one had given me any indication that I might need chemotherapy or any other therapy, for that matter. Once back in the conference room, my sister Janet and I waited and waited. We were there so long that we had to find a restroom. Something had come up and the doctor was an hour late. The financial representative for the office came in to talk about payment for subsequent visits and reiterated that a co-payment was a requirement each time I saw the doctor, even for continuing care, chemotherapy, and follow up care. Didn't anyone understand? *I'm just here for a consult.* The need to discuss the financial obligation seemed to be excessive. As a nurse, I understood that all medical care was expensive and the medical personnel needed to be paid but, this just seemed too much. They had obviously had problems in the past with clients paying their co-pay. I had breast cancer and my life was up in the air. How could anyone be concerned about finances right now? When the doctor finally arrived, he apologized for being so late. We certainly understood the medical profession and had nowhere else to be. That was not really true because I really would rather have been anywhere but here.

The doctor was charming, informative, and seemed to genuinely care about me. My sister thought I should have chemotherapy no matter what, but not me. He looked at my chart and the reports and started throwing out all the clinical trials because none of them applied to me. He was very upbeat and told me about a website sponsored by the Mayo Clinic that allowed you to input data and then gave you your chance of being alive in ten years. This was better known as the ten year survival rate. He took my data and filled it in and I had a 90% chance of being around in ten years. That sounded really good. My chances of being hit by a truck might have been better. We went over risks and the recommendations for treatment.

He suggested to me that I was really overcalling this and asked if I had thought about having a much less invasive lumpectomy (excision of just the tumor) and sentinel node biopsy, followed by radiation? Well no, not really. My left breast had betrayed me and I couldn't think of a reason to keep it. I knew that I actually wanted a bilateral mastectomy and I was pretty sure about the reconstruction. I did not care if this approach seemed too drastic. This was the only decision I could live with and be happy with. I certainly did not want to spend every waking hour worried about a recurrence. Then there was the dreaded tamoxifen. I had never heard anything good about this medication except that it did decrease recurrence by blocking estrogen from the tumors that loved and thrived on it. It would take away my libido, give me hot flashes, make me irritable and cause a slight increase in the occurrence of certain forms of cancer of the reproductive system. I had also resolved that since it would catapult me into menopause I would blow up to the size of a blimp. Of course, I thought of this, but not for long since this drug could potentially save my life or at least prolong it with a quality of life that was acceptable to me. I could not believe that I might need to take tamoxifen.

I was happy with my health and I did not want to change anything. The oncologist did say he was not a woman and could not possibly understand what I was going through. No he could not and I appreciated the fact that he could admit it. I did not really have cancer. I had it but it was gone. At least, this was what I believed. After all it was Stage I cancer with a T1 tumor. The doctor said the chance for axillary node metastasis was very low. I knew that I immediately put blinders on because I left feeling really good and not thinking I had a thing to worry about except surgery.

My sister had a lot of questions, and I did too. How would this diagnosis affect her, my niece, and my daughter and their future health? When we left after an hour or so and I decided that this had been a good encounter and I was feeling optimistic for the first time in days. Janet and I went out to lunch to celebrate. We both had veggie sandwiches. There seemed no better time than right now to start changing even the best dietary habits. I decided this optimism was good for my immune system and I needed everything in me to combat the spread of this disease. I started to visualize the battle inside me as good against evil. My family was here rallying around me. I had great friends and neighbors who encouraged me daily. How could anyone ask for more and how could I thank these people for everything they had done and planned to do?

The night after seeing the oncologist was a good one, finally. I slept fairly well. I was so relieved that chemotherapy would be unnecessary. Janet still insisted that I not rule it out. With or without lymph node involvement she felt chemotherapy was necessary. I did not agree at all. We could deal with that later. I felt the weight of the world begin to lift off my shoulders. For the first time I believed I might survive this. There were no guarantees in life but at least I had hope. The thought of hot flashes is not fun but I already had some occasionally. Hormone Replacement Therapy would not be an option for me so that dilemma was gone. The tumor was Her2/neu negative so treatment with herceptin would not be necessary. Receiving herceptin involved another year of therapy after all the others were complete. The pit in my stomach was not there and for the first time I actually felt hungry and I wanted to eat instead of just move my food all over the plate like a child. All I had to do was survive surgery and the biopsies and prove that the oncologist was correct. Oh, how wrong could I have been?

Chapter 4

Decisions

When I woke up early the next morning, with great relief and uncontainable excitement, I told Jim that I was going to be a breast cancer survivor. This was the first time I began to believe it. He was thrilled. Typically, Critical Care Nurses prepare for the worst. Today's doctor was the plastic surgeon again. She needed to take pictures, so I would have before and after pictures. This was definitely not what I had ever envisioned if I were to get before and after pictures. I looked at more pictures of other people who had gone through similar surgery. I was exhausted looking at more breasts than I ever cared to see. Not many people were Playboy models. I had no idea why I thought of that but I did. I hope I don't look old and flabby in the pictures. I had changed my mind about the reconstructive procedure I wanted. After much deliberation and a fair amount of research, I decided to have latissimus dorsi flaps and implants. The latissimus dorsi muscle ran down your back, in a matched set, one on either side, from shoulder to almost lower back. After the mastectomy, the surgery involved dissecting those muscles away from the underlying back muscles bringing a small amount of skin with the muscles (called a skin island), and tunneling them under the arm. From here they would be placed over saline breast implants to give a more natural feel and shape as well as provide an immediate reconstruction. I knew this decision would prolong surgery by at least four or five hours. That increased the risk of other complications like blood clots, infection, and pain. The rationale for this was the fact that I had a six year old daughter, Kate. She was my only daughter and I wanted to be around for a long time to see her grow up. I believed I would be on the road to recovery by Christmas so we could rejoice over the holidays. I also wanted to come out of surgery with breasts and not spend several months getting the implants inflated to then have to go back into surgery for permanent placement. I don't want my daughter to ever see me mutilated or not normal, at her young age. She had years of self esteem to establish and I did not want her to be affected by my scars and lack of breasts. I believed that opting for the inflatable implants would be hard to hide from her and might have affected how she viewed herself as a young teenager. She would have enough to deal with in the future just having a mother with breast cancer. I surely did not want to add to it with anything else that might affect her normal growth and development when she became an adolescent.

The surgeon and the plastic surgeon had a lot to do relative to the change in procedures and there was that never ending barrage of paperwork that needed to be completed. I felt really good about the team I assembled for my care. I just seemed to be spending all my time at doctor's appointments. There did not seem to be much time for anything else, after I got through seeing doctors. This cancer consumed my entire life and the life of my family. It might even be gone already, having chosen to have the excision biopsy. I interspersed the difficult days with appointments for me like haircuts and massages. When I went to the hair appointment I told the stylist about my cancer and had her give me a really short haircut so it would be easy to take care of when I came out of surgery. I knew it would be difficult to raise my arms and wash my hair. Or maybe I did not want so much hair to watch fall out if it was necessary to receive chemotherapy. The nagging doubts got worse over the last few weeks before surgery. My next two appointments were with the hospital and the general surgeon.

There was so much paperwork to ensure that insurance payments would be made. Sometimes I wanted to scream, "Hey, I am in here and I am a person with a potentially fatal disease. Does anyone really care about me?" I felt like everyone just wanted to be paid. I just wanted to wish this all away.

I was still waiting to wake up from the dream or maybe nightmare was a better term. It was still very surreal. I was able to get bits of sleep even when those little what ifs? invaded my sleep. My brother Harvey called to tell me that lumpectomy (wide excision but breast sparing procedure) with radiation and mastectomy with lymphadenectomy (removal of the entire breast and roughly one third of the lymph nodes under the arm) had the same survival rates. I knew this but it did not change my mind. I found it interesting that October was Breast Cancer Awareness Month and it was October so I had to deal with multiple articles in the newspapers and magazines with many suggestions. Everyone in my family wanted to weigh in with their suggestions as well. My dad, brother, and sister- in-law thought I was acting too drastically. I had *Wall Street Journal* articles and *US News and World Reports* articles.

I was a nurse and I knew what I wanted. I was certainly qualified to make the best decisions for my own health. No one persuaded me to do anything else no matter how many articles they sent to the contrary. I certainly did not want to keep the breast with the cancer and would like to get the other one removed so I wouldn't have to worry about a second tumor or a recurrence. I did not want to live the rest of my life worried constantly about each little lump. I felt like I would be carrying around a loaded pistol playing Russian roulette.

As I was researching my options for care, I became a sponsor of the virtual Race for the Cure. This was the annual run sponsored by the Susan G Komen Foundation, to raise money for breast cancer research. I knew I was not up to running, this year, but I believed in the cause and I surely liked the foundation and the percentage of money that actually went to the charity. Thanks to the Internet, I virtually sponsored someone from the comfort of my own home and slept the day of the race. It took place in Denver in a week or so. This year it had become very personal. Maybe next year I could run after this was all over. I wanted to be here a year from now and celebrate with the Race for the Cure. My emotions were all over the map right now. I still felt good about my surgical decisions. I hoped I was cured, but there was still that nagging doubt that jumped at me when my defenses were down. I cried a lot. My prayers started to center on chemotherapy. I didn't want it at all but my sister really believed it was necessary, regardless of the outcome of the surgery. Now I prayed that if I needed chemotherapy that I would have one positive lymph node because I knew that was the only way I would accept chemotherapy and all the side effects related to it. More scripture appeared in my box at my door. These kind gestures certainly helped me keep the faith while the world seemed to be falling down around me.

Knowing what lay ahead, as it got later in October, I tried to get as much of my holiday shopping done as possible. I already knew a few things that I wanted to get and I raced out to various stores to purchase them and have them ready. I had no idea what the future held but I did know that recovering from major surgery took about six weeks. I could do a lot of shopping on line and through catalogs. For my sanity I loved to go to the mall because I liked to window shop. I preferred to relax just wandering around the stores but right now I was on a mission. I also knew that I would not feel much like shopping until almost Christmas and that was only if I did not need further treatment. If I needed more treatment like chemotherapy I might never leave the house again to shop this season. Even shopping now was pretty difficult and that neon sign that I believed followed me was hanging around my neck. I looked at everyone and wondered if they were facing trials like I was. I also wondered how many more years I would have to shop like this. I loved to get out before the crowds and really give gifts a lot of thought. I also could not imagine how many people might know that I had cancer and feel really sorry for me. I did not want to be an object of pity. This was really very egocentric of me to think that people I didn't know were concerned about anything that I did. For some reason I believed that everyone I saw knew that I had cancer and felt sorry for me. This was fairly irrational and self-centered but I could not shake the feeling.

My niece was leaving for the Avon 3-day Breast Cancer Walk in Malibu, California to walk it with friends with whom she went to school. A month ago, before my diagnosis, when she began collecting pledges, she put a brief message on the website about why she felt strongly about raising money for Breast Cancer research. Her paragraph included something about how although for her, a close family member or friend had never been diagnosed with breast cancer she believed in the cause. Things changed very quickly since her decision was made and I was touched that she walked for me now. My niece was about half way between my sister's age and mine so I felt like I helped raise her. She felt very much like a sister to me. Of course I cried at her thoughtfulness, too.

My sister had a friend from childhood who was running the Race for the Cure in Atlanta. I knew her quite well also. She later sent me a picture of the placard on the back of her running shirt because she also ran for me. The race allowed you to run in memory of a person or in celebration of one who was fighting or a survivor. I wasn't sure which I was going to be but there was my name pinned to her back. It read, *In Celebration of Joannie Yeash*. I cried every time I looked at the picture.

Six days before my surgery as I worked out on my elliptical trainer, which I was still doing several times a week, I was sweating and sobbing. I kept up the workouts because I knew there would be several weeks after surgery that I would not be allowed to exercise. I was suddenly overcome by fear and was emotionally feeling control slip away. At that moment I realized that if something happened to me in surgery and I never woke up, my family was ill-equipped to handle any of our affairs. I paid all the bills, made most of the financial decisions, knew where all the important documents were, paid for Jerred's (my oldest son) college tuition, and I took care of all these things for my dad as well. How would my family manage? What would I say to them if I knew I would not be coming out of surgery? I kept crying and sweating but decided when I was done to start my own Kick the Bucket file. In my family this was affectionately known as the KTB. My dad has a KTB file. I think he coined the name. I would be forever grateful for his insight in preparing this, years before it was necessary, as would my sister and brother. My mother had one that my dad wrote for her. It was invaluable after her death. It was organized and helped us stay on task and accomplish all the necessary things without losing focus on what we were doing during our time of grieving. It also helped us to identify areas that needed revision. Once I resolved that I needed to do this for peace of mind, I was able to function and get on with the day. I took care of some medical billing issues with my dad and then came home to mow the lawn.

It was a beautiful autumn day and the sunshine and fresh air were good for me. I thought it might be the last time I would mow the lawn since the site of the excision biopsy hurt a bit while I pushed the mower. I was sure that the lengthier surgery would cause even more discomfort and mowing the lawn just did not seem like something I would be able to do or want to do after surgery, at least not right away. It was a small job that made me feel very normal, if only for a brief period of time.

Justin's soccer team lost their play-off game last night, five days before my surgery, so the season was over. Ryan finished soccer last week as well. The timing of my surgery seemed good because everyone would be finished with their sports so Ryan would be available to drive his siblings where they needed to go, like Kate's dance class and basketball practice. He was not looking forward to his carpooling duties, but I relied on him a lot. Justin's marching band would be finished soon. Not that I wanted the kids to lose or place very low but I was just not prepared to go on with any more competitions. There had been many late nights and now my biggest concern was keeping everyone healthy so that I could stay healthy for surgery. I started to increase my vitamin intake to include magnesium, selenium, beta-carotene and vitamin C. I wanted my immune system to be functioning at its maximum capacity. I taught myself to meditate and use visualization to boost my immune system to the best of my abilities. I had not perfected either, because I wanted to meditate with prayer and I did not like the good cell /bad cell visualization I started on other's recommendations. I revised this as I went along with the learning process. I was just thankful to know how to visualize and had the time to spend perfecting it.

I finally sat down to work on my KTB file. This was not an easy task, particularly through the tears which I could not stop. I carefully wrote out the location of important documents and who the important contact people were. I included who I wanted told of my death, should it occur. That was not something I had ever contemplated. It really made me think about my life and who would care if I was gone. I included information on all of the accounts we had and where they were located. I never realized the information that I had and about which Jim had no idea. Thank goodness we had the good sense to write a will a few years ago that established a trust for the kids. I really could not deal with that right now. I just hoped the lawyer and the trust account executive could get Jim through all this if the need arose. He was a wonderful doctor, husband, and father, but had never paid much attention to the details of our financial planning or insurance. I hurried through the creation of this document but I hoped I would have plenty of time to revise it over the course of the rest of my life. I also had put a survivor benefit plan into effect through my army retirement, primarily for the kids, that should I die before I reach the age of sixty; the family would receive a monthly check. I spent 21 years in the army and army reserve as a nurse, caring for people like me and teaching others how to be a nurse and I would like my family to reap some benefit from that if I did not live to retirement age myself. It might help offset childcare fees and college tuition. I realized now how unprepared we were for the death of either Jim or me. This diagnosis had certainly forced me to consider these possibilities. Jim was not very thrilled to be forced to deal with them, as I think he looked upon my efforts as giving up and he wanted to stay totally optimistic. I looked at it as being prepared.

I wondered if everyone who faced surgery and cancer contemplated these issues. I felt a bit obsessive-compulsive. Next I wrote a note to each of my kids and my husband. If I thought the KTB proved to be tough and I had not quit crying, writing letters to my loved ones was no easier. What do you say to the people most important in your life when they varied in age from 6-60? Not to mention my dad at 86. I couldn't even write anything for him. He was my hero and the person who had been there for me my whole life. He and my mom taught me morals, ethics, integrity, and honor. Duty, honor, and country were ingrained in our soul and we did not lie, cheat, or steal nor tolerate those who did. If it sounded militaristic, it should because that was the US Military Academy's honor code and that was my honor code as well.

It wasn't always easy but my dad was always there. He was often brusque, but my mom could always temper him a bit. He was supposed to die first not me. That was the natural order of things. I hoped he knew how much I loved him because there was no way I could put it into words. With the rest of the family, I tried to put my thoughts into the written word. I cannot begin to tell them everything I thought right then but it was a start. I hoped I had told all of them how wonderful they were. I knew that I had not because it was so hard and now I burst into tears when I tried to tell them anything. Why did we wait so long to tell the important people in our lives what they meant to us? If I survived this surgery, I would try to change that. I wrote each family member a note on the computer but I could not even bring myself to tell anyone that they were there. I finally told my friend Geri and my sister the day of surgery about the documents. They didn't really want to hear it, because it forced them to accept reality and our absolute vulnerability, but someone needed to know where this information could be found. I did not want to tell Jim because I didn't want him to think I was giving up. During the weeks before surgery I wrote in a journal every day so that I could keep my thoughts straight. Events occurred so fast and many were having a huge impact on my life and how I lived it. I did not want to forget one minute of this journey.

About a week before surgery the High School had parent-teacher conferences and I wanted to go see how Ryan (age 17) and Justin (age 15) were doing. These were very time consuming and tedious because a lot of time was spent standing in line and waiting. It's easier if both Jim and I went, since we have two kids and two sets of teachers. However, I tried to see all the teachers during one session since I had no idea if Jim could attend the next day. I had not spent much time out in public because I had been so busy with appointments seeing all the doctors. I had not shared my health information with anyone except those I called *the inner circle*. The inner circle were those friends who were very close to me and my family. I gave my neighbor, Nancy, permission to tell a few people because she wanted to get prayers started. As I stood around looking at all the people at these conferences I wondered if they could possibly know what I was going through. I wished it was not me who was going through this but I sure would not wish it on any one else either. In my mind I was sure people were staring at me and could somehow tell that I had cancer. I wondered if I would ever feel normal again. My life had been forever changed and soon my body would be forever changed. I kept moving along with the conferences and hoped I would not stand around with too much time to think. I saw both boys' teachers who were there and I was pleased. If Jim got a chance to go, he would only have one or two teachers to meet. As I walked out of the gym and down the hall I saw one of the other soccer moms selling school sport's clothing for fundraising. I sat down briefly and talked to her. I had no idea what possessed me to tell her about the situation. Her daughter and Justin were really good friends and I think I just wanted him to have her support. The mom was also a nurse and I had gone to first aid training with her a few years earlier. Whatever the reason, I told her that I had breast cancer and I would be having a bilateral mastectomy and reconstruction in a week. Because of her nursing background, I explained a little more about the prognosis to her and told her it looked really good but that I was not willing to take any chances. I knew I took her totally by surprise since I had seen her at several soccer games and never mentioned a thing to her. Certainly, now the word may begin to get around, but I did not want to be an object of pity.

My kid's activities finally wound down. I finished my last letter to my family and I had five days until surgery. It all seemed very morbid but I felt like it was necessary. I did not want anyone to forget me. That was probably the hardest thing for me to deal with. Kate was only six. She might not remember me. My sister-in-law Kitty was nine when her mother died from breast cancer and she had only vague memories of her mother and her younger sister and brother who were six and three years old at that time remember nothing. I wished my children were older or I was older. I was feeling like I had not been the best wife and mother. I thought I could have done much better. I would certainly work on that if I got through this. My transition from working woman to stay at home mom had been so hard. That all seemed fairly trivial in retrospect, but not at the time. I wanted no unfinished business before surgery. I relaxed as much as possible for the next few days before surgery and spent time with my family. Surgery approached quickly and I needed it to be over to find peace. What kind of a legacy have I left and what would I be remembered for? These were difficult questions to deal with and most people had more than several weeks or days to deal with them. I needed to take a good look at this some time soon.

Two days before my surgery my dearest friends took me to dinner. The group included neighbors Nancy, Lisa and her mom, Sue, who had breast cancer, Nanette, Terri, Suzi, Katy, and Amy. It was great fun and a wonderful way to get my mind off the impending surgery. These friends had been praying for me and leaving notes of inspiration. They were extremely supportive and were not afraid to jump in with both feet. I learned that when people found out you were really sick, they either pulled away because they cannot deal with their own mortality, or they have come to terms with that and were able to be of immense help and comfort. We all reached these stages at different times and it did not make anyone more or less a better friend. It lives and what they had the endurance to face. Some of us are forced to mature faster than others.

At dinner Nancy asked me what I saw in this experience that let me know that God was there. At first I was speechless because like most people going through cancer, you asked God constantly why this was happening. You even questioned whether He was still there. Then you questioned how good you really were as a Christian and what you did wrong in your life that caused you to have a potentially fatal disease. I asked myself these questions often. I never thought about how God might be working in my life. After I thought briefly my answer was "look around the table." Looking at these wonderful friends and the way they touch peoples' lives was my proof that God was there. I cried with these people and rejoiced with these people. We prayed together and mourned together. We were raising our children together and growing older together. I hoped that they would always remember me and never forget to have their yearly mammograms and do their monthly breast self examinations. That was God working through me to help save lives. As a registered nurse I was always involved in health teaching. This was perhaps my most important life lesson. I felt good to have any influence of this magnitude on any life I touched. That was my passion at this moment in my life. I knew that every experience allowed us to grow deeper in our faith and I was just beginning my cancer adventure. I felt in my heart that it would be a difficult one, with many obstacles. I would certainly be glad when my first hurdle, surgery, was over. My friends Nancy and Suzi prayed with me that night after dinner. We cried a lot. But there was a peace that came through prayer and I had thousands of people around the country praying with me and for me. Every now and then I felt a fleeting moment of peace when I was overwhelmed with love and I was sure that it was the result of many prayers coming my way from all over the country.

Again my sleep was suffering and I had resorted to taking sleeping pills every night along with a mild tranquilizer. I thought I needed to be well rested to stay healthy, and I surely could not stay healthy if I was up all night ruminating about this cancer. I was not a drug addict but I was concerned about taking the medications. Thankfully, my oncologist assured me that I was normal in my temporary need for sleep and anti-anxiety aids. He explained that many cancer patients needed these types of medications for short periods of time.

My sister and my friend Geri came in the day before surgery, October 23. Geri took several days off work to be with me. I was so thankful and blessed to be surrounded by so much love. My forces massed and all of my support systems would soon be in place. It was almost like a battle plan. The last things I did before my day of surgery was get a massage and then spend some time with Kate doing a manicure and pedicure for her. She loved to get her nails done and I wanted her to have good memories of our time together before I left for the hospital. I've seen the same massage therapist for almost ten years. She's enlightened me with all sorts of alternative medicine information through the years as well as provided me with much needed stress relief. I gave her a hug before I left and got a little teary. My mother-in-law was here for love and support for the kids and to help them get through any rough times they had.

Janet spent the night with my dad at his apartment since we thought he needed some support, too. Geri was staying here with us. I made her take some before photos of my profile with my old breasts. I was fully clothed but it was hard to know they would be gone in 24 hours. I needed to do something to remember this occasion. It was actually a pretty funny thing to do and my family thought I was nuts. We had a few laughs as a result of my request and we all needed the relief that a few minutes of giggling and laughter gave us.

Chapter 5

Surgery

October 24th, the day of surgery arrived. I felt confident with the team of surgeons that I had so carefully assembled. I was scared to death and hungry. I tried to get the kids off to school just like normal. I felt weepy but I tried to be strong so they would not know how frightened I really was. The morning dragged by. Of course I couldn't eat anything or drink anything. Nancy came over and sat with us as we all stared into space. We tried to make small talk and joked a little bit. I knew the situation was difficult for all of us and I was grateful not to be alone. I never knew how hard it was to wait until afternoon for surgery. All my surgery rotations as a student started at about 5:30 am. I was never with anyone late in the day. After several painfully slow hours and a shower, we finally left for the hospital.

I entered the pre-operative area around 11:00 am after another endless paperwork shuffle necessary for any surgery or hospitalization. I looked like a deer in the oncoming headlights of a car at night, paralyzed with fear.

All the medical and nursing knowledge I had, seemed at this moment, to be useless. I had been the comforter for my patients, my husband, and my family when they needed it, but this role was very hard. I needed comforting but I had no idea how to ask for it because I was a healthcare professional and people thought I knew everything and did not need comforting or reassuring. I wanted to be out of touch and relax. Of course I had to be alert to sign all the paperwork. My sister Janet and my husband Jim were with me in pre-op. Janet asked all the right questions. I tried to keep up small talk with the nurses and my family. I saw a lot of folks I knew. My neighbors were anesthesiologists and surgeons. They all seemed to be there that day. There was a steady stream of people passing by the end of my bed. Some I knew and some I had never seen before. The room was quite cramped and I felt a bit like I was on display. I knew they felt sorry for me. I hated that, but I would feel sorry for me too if I were them. It was an endless series of introductions as my sister began to meet my surgical team. The plastic surgeon arrived and met Janet. The general surgeon had not yet arrived.

The nurses started my intravenous line. They also put on little wraps around the calves of my legs that inflated and deflated to maintain circulation to my lower extremities, to reduce my chances of getting blood clots. I asked my neighbor the anesthesiologist if he would be doing my surgery. He said no, that I was getting the senior partner in the group. Apparently my surgery today was quite a big deal. I was honored. This man had also done the spinal anesthesia when I had a tubal ligation after Kate was born. I thought he was great. I didn't remember getting poked with the spinal needle but I was awake for the procedure. I was up and about in a very short time after the tubal ligation. I knew this time would be different.

I was terribly frightened of general anesthesia. This was definitely one of those times when knowing anything was too much. I remembered all the patients that I had been with when they were intubated and I could also remember a lot of the crass jokes during long cases in the Operating Room. One woman in particular that I remembered had one breast that was too big and one that was too small. I observed her surgery and I hated the way the plastic surgeons joked about her breasts as they performed her surgery. Too much about breasts as far as I was concerned. I did not want anyone telling jokes about me while I was under anesthesia.

This surgery would be lengthy. The double mastectomy would take 1-2 hours and the reconstruction would take another 4 hours. So six hours seemed like an eternity. Would I wake up in the middle? Would I feel any pain? Would they be able to keep my blood pressure up? Would they forget to breathe for me? Most of all would I wake up with my Benign Paroxysmal Positional Vertigo? I kept telling them to make sure they medicated me for nausea because when BPPV struck it did so with a vengeance. Nausea and vomiting followed immediately. I didn't know if it was a result of many years of high impact exercise (running) or if the maneuvers my massage therapist did with my neck set it off, I just knew if I woke up with it, watch out. I also knew that for the plastic surgeon to do the reconstruction, I would be flipped over from front to back a few times as well as lifted to the sitting position. Remember breasts draped and she wanted to get it just right. To do that she had to get gravity working for her by having me sit up and drawing on me with a nice purple pen to mark her surgical areas. I also knew that in order for the anesthesiologist to intubate me that he would have to hyper-extend my neck. The general surgeon had the best job. Take the breasts off and go home.

My next slightly strange concern was that my period was late and I was afraid I would start bleeding on the operating room table and the staff would think I was hemorrhaging. She assured me that happened all the time and they were well prepared for it. Oh my, what had I ever done in my life to deserve having to go through this? I knew that my family would have a much harder time with surgery than I would. After all, I would be asleep and at least I thought I would not notice the passage of time. If it was like labor with my children I was conscious of every minute but I knew that under a general anesthetic you were not awake and did not notice the passage of time, at least I hoped I would not. The family would have to wait long agonizing hours. I told them all to go home for several hours but I really did not think they would do that. Jim could be reached on a pager and Janet could make decisions if he was not there. My dad could not deal with the stress of the hospital so I made him stay home. What anyone actually did I would not know about until after the surgery since I would be under the general anesthetic and thankfully so.

Two of the kids were to perform in music concerts on the same night so we decided Geri and Grandma Yeash would go to Kate's concert and Jim would go to Justin's Jazz Band Concert. Both were taking place within half a mile of the hospital. Janet stayed in the waiting room. I wanted the family to have something to do beside worry about me all day.

All of my extremities were freezing in the pre-op area so the nurses kept bringing me more warm blankets, but I could not seem to get warm. I visualized a warm beach and the sun and the water as it lapped against the shore. I finally got sedation by intravenous line which made me feel calmer. Anna from the operating room came out to talk to me. She was the last person in the series who needed to talk to me or ask questions. We talked briefly and it was time to be wheeled back into the operating room. The one thing she said to me was that people never remembered the operating room staff. I made a point right then that I would not forget her. Amazingly I was not crying at all now. It must be the medication. Janet and Jim both gave me a kiss. I did not want to say good-bye, just see you later. I said a prayer and asked God to get me through this and get my family through this. He knew what was in my heart, so I could be brief. I gave Jim the little angel medal I had been holding since I got to the hospital. It was a gift from our friend Melissa.

It was 12:30 pm, right on time. The activity was bustling. The OR (operating room) was freezing but they assured me that as soon as I got moved onto the bed in the OR they would warm me up. Why was it always so cold? I was never cold in the OR as a student. The OR seemed huge and I was under an enormous light. The plastic surgeon was already in the room making sure that my implants arrived and worked. She checked for leaks and obvious problems.   So much of what she did was pure art. I spent as much time as I could examining my surroundings and trying to commit them to memory. There were many cabinets of storage space, but there was still a lot of equipment, I noticed, just sitting around the room. The people in there were just going about their jobs very efficiently. Soon there would be even more people in there. Everyone was so busy except me. I wanted to jump up and scream but I did not know what I would scream. I was still so terribly cold. Maybe they wanted me to be hypothermic (for my body temperature to be low). I saw a little window which I thought was nice. A little sunshine was good. There was music playing through the speakers from somewhere. It was a pop radio station. I might have chosen classical but didn't have any voice in the decision. I thought I might like to observe more but the anesthesiologist was already there, so they strapped each arm down at a right angle from my body and they strapped my feet together. I did not like that at all. My body was in the shape of a cross. It was hard not to think of the crucifixion in this position. I thought this was to keep me from falling off the very narrow bed. I said little prayers to God, like don't desert me now and please stay with me. I had a little conversation with God while I tried to relax. I attempted to take all my surroundings in as they got me ready for surgery but I was fairly sleepy now. It was easier to shut my eyes and relax. The anesthesiologist briefly spoke to me and then the mask loomed over me like a huge boulder ready to fall at any moment. It came down over my nose and mouth. I think he said goodnight. I remembered nothing else.

The first few minutes the staff prepared me for surgery. They positioned me and then removed all the bedding from the waist up. They would then clean the surgical site with anti- microbial soap to prevent infection. Circular incisions were made on each breast around the nipple and areola. The skin and areola complex were then removed. The general surgeon removed both breasts sparing as much of the skin that is left to facilitate the reconstruction process. I envisioned this as having my breast tissue scooped out like ice cream with an ice cream scoop. I was sure it was more scientific than that. The amount of skin removed from the left breast was a bit more than the right breast because not only was all breast tissue removed, but the surgeon also had to reach toward my axilla (arm pit) and removed lymph nodes. It was done a bit blindly and they were never sure exactly how many nodes they removed until after the pathology report was received. This process took about an hour.

The plastic surgeon replaced the general surgeon and began the reconstruction. This involved estimating the amount of skin and muscle that would be needed so it was just enough to cover the implant. Earlier she had drawn purple lines on my back to give her an idea where to make the large incisions necessary to dissect the latisimus dorsi muscle on both my right and left sides. This involved being flipped from my front to my back as well as on my sides several times as well as being brought to a sitting position to visualize the effect of gravity on the tissue. Once the latisimus muscle and a round skin island were dissected, they were tunneled under the skin under my arm and brought to the correct position at the site of each breast. The implant was positioned with the top under my pectoralis muscle and then the latisimus was placed over the implant for a more natural looking breast. I remembered thinking how large the implant was when I was at my first consultation but was reassured at how large the actual breast pocket was, extending from just under the clavicle (collarbone) to almost the tip of the sternum (breastbone). Finally using very small stitches the skin islands were sewed into place on top of each breast. Bandages were applied after cleaning the surgical site. Once again I was covered with warm blankets and taken to the Recovery Room until I awakened enough to be taken to a hospital room.

Part 2

Chapter 6

Recovery

Suddenly I began to hear voices calling to me. Joan are you awake? We're taking you to your room now. Surgery was done. I don't even remember being in the recovery room but I'm sure I was there for awhile. I saw lights, bright lights and I felt the gurney moving down the hall. I wondered what people with near death experiences saw. I could tell when we got to the elevator because the bump getting on to the elevator caused some pain. I drifted off again and then I was in my room. There was all sorts of commotion. Everyone asked if I was nauseated. I couldn't seem to open my mouth but I shook my head no I was not nauseated. I heard people talking. The plastic surgeon told me it was all over and I had done really well. Halleluiah, I had made it through surgery. Thank you heavenly Father for letting me still be here. "Joan, Nancy is here to see if you are out of surgery yet?" She should be at the concert. I pointed to my arm where my watch should be. Jim told me that it was 10:00pm. I seemed only to be able to communicate in sign language. I couldn't talk yet. Someone asked me again if I was nauseated or in pain. I think it was the plastic surgeon. All I could do was draw the letter N with my hand in the air. Jim asked if that meant nausea. I shook my head yes. Actually I remembered not really having any idea if I was nauseated or in pain. He wondered why I kept signing everything and I shrugged my shoulders. Doing that hurt a lot. I didn't even think my eyes were open yet and if they were I couldn't see anything. I knew that surgery had lasted nine and a half hours! Of course I calculated in my head because I still could not seem to form words or ask questions with my mouth. Nancy went home after she knew surgery had gone well. I think I waved at her. I was pretty sure I waved at someone. She had taken the kids home from the concert and come back. Wow, what a friend. It was so late at night. The plastic surgeon told me I had great lats (latissimus dorsi muscles) and the surgery went really well. I think she told me that already but I could not remember very well. Everyone laughed about my great lats except me. I hurt all over. In fact I felt like I had been hit by a car. My great lats were not where they were supposed to be anymore and I was frightened of what was yet to come.

Everyone was obsessed with the nausea. According to the plastic surgeon I received multiple doses of anti-nausea medications. They paid attention to me and I felt no positional vertigo and I was ecstatic that the medical personnel had listened to me and heeded my advice. I think I scared them by telling them about all the vomiting. The nursing staff explained to me I had patient controlled analgesia and I had to push the button when I had pain in order to dose myself with pain medication. I could do that. I pushed the button right away. No one else was allowed to push the button for me. The dispenser was filled with dilaudid since I refused morphine, the more common drug for patient controlled analgesia (pain control). I made that really clear before the surgery. I had a patient once, when I was a new nurse in the army, who was a general surgeon having orthopedic surgery and I remembered him telling me, "L-T (for lieutenant), this morphine is awful. It doesn't take away the pain; it just makes me unable to tell you how bad the (expletive) pain really is." That was 25 years ago and I have never forgotten his words. The night after my surgery was a blur but at least I was able to finally talk. I didn't really remember everyone leaving. Jim had gone home as had my plastic surgeon. Janet stayed with me. There was quite a commotion as she tried to put her bed up because she couldn't quite get it up and made quite a racket before she finally called the nursing personnel for help with it. I was glad to have some one there because I felt groggy and I hurt everywhere and I thought I would be very afraid to stay alone in my groggy state.

After getting an epidural block during the birth of my fifth child, I had been left alone unable to move anything below my waist. I kept feeling like I was going to pass out but I was lying down. My blood pressure kept dropping and I had to keep positioning the bed so I got enough blood to my brain. I spent four hours all by myself doing that before someone finally came in to check on me. It had been an awful feeling. I had five children and I was a nurse, therefore, the tendency was to assume that we knew everything. Nothing could be further from the truth. Needless to say, Janet's presence was a tremendous comfort to me.

There were four drains in my back and a huge dressing over my breasts. The dressing I could see but not the drains. I felt like I had a watermelon on my chest. I sure hoped the new breasts were not that big. I'll deal with that later as I was just too tired right now. Thankfully I had a Foley catheter draining my bladder, so I won't have to get up and go to the bathroom. I didn't really want that either but the length of the surgery dictated its necessity. I dozed on and off all night. My sister woke up every time I moved. Yes I was still OK, but when I fell asleep I forget the pain medicine so each time I awakened I was in excruciating pain. The pain was from the donor site on my back not the mastectomy and reconstruction site. Those darned drains were painful, too. I finally found out where they were when I moved around and landed on them. I felt tight all over; of course my entire trunk was bandaged with something. There was a lot of pain. I really got the hang of this patient controlled analgesia. Someone forgot to send me the memo on how badly your body hurts after surgery. I sure appreciated what my patients had gone through over the years. Then there was coughing and deep breathing. I already felt my lungs rattle from the accumulated mucus which resulted from being in the same position on my back for a long period of time. I tried my hardest to cough because I sure did not want to develop pneumonia. This first night, the nursing staff hovered over me. Of course I was nauseous from the pain medication and had to keep asking for anti-nausea medicine and they measured the output from the drains hourly. Somewhere in there I managed to sleep. It seemed that whatever did not hurt then was numb. That was an odd sensation.

At 5:00 am someone from the lab came into the room to draw blood. I had done this hundreds of times, but for the life of me, I could not figure out why it could not be drawn at a more civilized 7:30 or 8:00 am. I must have dozed again because the next time I woke up, it was daylight. I was still there and survived the night. I was hungry too. Of course I can't have anything to eat until the doctor's saw me. Luckily they rounded early. First the general surgeon arrived. She seemed really upbeat and told me things had gone well. I asked if she saw anything suspicious when they removed the breast tissue. She said no, everything looked fine and they saw nothing suspicious, at least grossly speaking. She did not look at my breasts under a microscope. It looked like I was cancer free. I felt a little more optimistic, but I had heard this all before so my guard was up, to say the least. The pathology tests would be back on Monday since there's another weekend to contend with. I really needed to not schedule surgeries on Thursdays. Since the cancer was on the left side, they had also performed a lymph node dissection on that side. It did not seem too scientific. They just reached up and grabbed a bunch of tissue which was largely fat and included about a third of the lymph nodes from under the arm. There was also a nerve imbedded in the fat so there was a lot of numbness postoperatively. That might go away or last forever. That arm on the left was also at risk for lymphedema. This is a condition that causes swelling of the arm as a result of lymph not being drained from the arm due to the lack of one third of the lymph nods. It could be fairly minor or really severe and no one was quite sure who might develop this problem or what exactly caused some people to develop it and some people not to develop it.

For the rest of my life, no blood should be drawn from my left arm, blood pressures should not be taken on that side, and I should not have any injections in my left arm. You wanted to avoid anything that could cause an infection or restrict blood flow to the arm. As I looked down, there was my IV line in my left hand, a little red, swollen, and painful. I might already be a statistic. Some people go as far as to say not to wear a watch or jewelry on the affected side either. That would be hard. I can't even fit my wedding and engagement rings on the other ring finger. Seemed like a silly thing to worry about. I thought I would get a medic alert bracelet, warning of the potential for lymphedema. I could use it as a teaching tool as well as have it as a precaution. This was the first of the permanent changes in my life.

My biggest concern however, was how to shave under that affected arm. From my research it was suggested that you not use a safety razor. I just hated to give up my safety razor for an electric one. They just never worked well enough. It's amazing what cropped up as an annoyance as you came out of surgery.

I received permission to eat clear liquids and the Jell-O tasted surprisingly good. I would rather have had an omelet. The worst thing I could imagine would be to get a paralytic ileus from eating too soon or too much so I'm fairly content to eat a lot of jello and drink clear liquids. When you were under general anesthetic, everything is paralyzed including your intestines. If you started to eat before your intestines were able to move food through, it just sat in the intestines like a brick, causing nausea and vomiting.

I finally got up the nerve and looked under my bandages when the plastic surgeon came. Actually, my plastic surgeon was so excited she wanted me to look. I had two breast mounds and they looked huge, and just like they had a bull's eye right in the center of each one. Both breasts had been scooped out, the nipples removed, and a circle of skin called a skin island had been brought around from my back along with the latisimus dorsi muscle. It was very exciting, or so I kept telling myself. The plastic surgeon was certainly excited and I felt badly that I could not join in her exuberance. With all the bandaging I felt like a football lineman. I was thankful I saw two breasts and not two flat areas without breasts. I'm glad I decided on an immediate reconstruction. Even the suture lines looked great already. The stitches were so tiny that they almost disappeared. The huge bandages masked the large incisions from where my latisimus dorsi muscles and skin were taken. Maybe it was best not to see them just yet but, my back sure felt tight. The drains leaked around their insertion sites so it was a bit damp too. Every time I moved I felt fluid oozing out of the holes for the drains. Oh well, that's why they make those funny blue disposable pads for beds called chux; the ones that never worked when you wanted them to. At least with all my patients I seemed to be changing entire beds because the blue pads were not useful. They just stuck to patients.

I was one day out from the surgery and I felt nauseous still from the pain medication and the nurses kept giving me medicine for the nausea. I had 5000 cc of urine output. Everyone was astounded. I always knew I drank a lot. The catheter was driving me crazy so I had it pulled out by late afternoon. Not the smartest time to have it removed since it's almost bedtime. Just having the catheter stay in increases the chance for a urinary tract infection and I had all I needed to deal with right now. After a catheter is removed one has a lot of urgency and it takes several trips to the toilet before the plumbing is functioning properly. Preferably night is not be the time to deal with this. I would never have discontinued a catheter on a patient at night. I managed to get my kidneys working before late that night and even managed to get in and out of bed but it was not very comfortable. Janet was still there to help. That night I think we both slept better but I still felt strange. I was interrupted a lot during the night and had to give myself pain medication every time I woke up. Then of course, I also requested anti-nausea medication to treat the nausea caused by the pain medication. It was quite a vicious cycle. The next day was Saturday and Janet had to leave early Sunday and would not be staying with me that night. The anticipation of her departure made me really teary. Geri volunteered to stay but I decided I would try this on my own.

Today I was able to eat regular meals but I woke up nauseous and woozy. Though I could eat I did not feel like it. I was so disappointed and I felt like I was not making any progress.

Both surgeons came in this morning too. The general surgeon turned me over to the plastic surgeon for the rest of my care. Her part was done. Just that quickly my breasts were gone. Those were the breasts I waited anxiously for as a twelve year old and then complained about because I was never very well endowed. Those were also the breasts that grew with every pregnancy which I loved. I was well endowed during pregnancies and while breast feeding. Those were also the breasts that nourished each of my beautiful little babies. The bond between a nursing mother and newborn is instant and I fell in love even more with the babies as I breast fed them. They provided life and they produced the milk that may have saved the life of my third son, Justin. The pediatrician told me when he had an infection in his blood, in Belgium, at five weeks old that if I had not been breast feeding he might not have had enough antibodies to fight the massive infection. Now, my breasts were gone.

Sure I had replaced them, but the new ones had no feeling and never would. A part of me was gone forever and to some extent I had to mourn that loss. It seemed odd that the part of me I was anxious to get rid of, because of the cancer, now caused me so many tears. Maybe it's just the hospital and the pain and that awful pain medication.

Since I was so woozy on the dilaudid, the doctor decided to switch me to vicodin which was given as a pill by mouth every three hours. My intravenous line became infected and painful, so it had to be moved to another location. Now I had a huge painful left wrist. I saw that coming yesterday. That can't be good for my already compromised left arm. I was the only one to worry. Once I started the vicodin, I took it every three hours without fail. My eyes had a hard time focusing but I thought it must be the drugs and anesthesia.

I had a seemingly steady stream of visitors and I sort of felt like I was not really there. I felt like I was watching myself in a movie. But I knew that I was talking to them. My neck got sore from following the visitors around the room. Everyone was very happy that there was no sign of cancer but I just could not seem to relax. I was in pain. Moving was difficult. I couldn't just grab the bedrails and pull myself up because parts of my back muscles were now nonfunctional. Jim came in and out all day in between keeping some degree of normalcy for the rest of the family. Janet was a life saver and when she was not there Geri was there to pick up the slack. What would I have done without them?

I decided to go outside the hospital to walk around while Geri was there to go with me. Despite my discomfort I knew it would be good to go outside for a walk. Every nurse knew that you wanted to get patients walking as soon as possible after surgery. We looked at the new construction and walked through the parking lot. It felt great to be out on a beautiful fall day. Janet drove back while we were walking and was happy to see me out. We all sat in front of the hospital until the shade made it too chilly. I hardly saw the nurses except when I called for more pain medicine. I must have become quite the nuisance, because from my experience, that was when nurses tried to avoid you. When my parents had been hospitalized over the past few years, they were quite difficult to take care of and became quite demanding. The staff would avoid answering their requests. It seemed like much ado about nothing when Janet and Geri or Jim were there so constantly, but as soon as they left I was horribly lonely. I was sad and had lost part of my body and it was just an everyday occurrence to the staff.

I was tired and nauseated but Janet decided I was going to take a shower. One drain had been pulled out so I was down to three. A shower would feel really good and Janet had it all planned. She wrapped me in an intricate series of garbage bags so none of the bandages got wet. One went over my head and I looked ridiculous. She then decided to take off her shirt so it didn't get wet. She plopped me on the seat in the shower and pulled down the hand sprayer. The water was warm and nothing had ever felt so good. She soaped me up and shampooed my hair. That felt great too. All I had to do was hold the garbage bags on. As we worked down to my feet I could get rid of the bags because they were hot and sticky and felt like a steam room. We looked a sight and we both had a good laugh over this event; she with no shirt on and me covered with garbage bags. This was a great idea since I started to smell after two days with no shower. When I was clean, I felt as good as I had since before the surgery.

We ordered dinner together. The meal sounded good when I ordered but when it got there I could barely eat. I struggled through with what I could swallow. I was nauseous again. Janet left to bring my dad back for a brief visit. I just wanted to cry and scream but I could not do that in front of all these people. I felt like I was losing my mind. I was nauseous and was sure I would throw up but I felt better than before. I said goodbye to Janet and she took dad home and I slowly got ready for bed. I never had this much time to myself, it's a shame I felt so awful. I got more pain medicine and went to bed. I was so very nauseous but I tried to breathe through it and get some sleep. I heard the stupid clock in my room tick tocking. Why would anyone put such a noisy clock in a hospital room? If I could I would climb up and take it down and hide it under a pillow. Seemingly no one checked on me all night. I did get a little sleep, more than the two previous nights anyway, despite a fair amount of commotion out in the hall. The man in the room next to me came in with pneumonia and never quit calling out for the nurses and coughing, all night. I wanted to go in there and suction out his lungs so he and I could both get some rest.

By the time I woke up I knew Janet's plane had left and I felt really yucky. That was not a very medical term but it described it well. I tried to order food, but nothing sounded good. I tried to eat some granola and yogurt but I only managed a few bites. Then I decided to take a walk by myself. I thought I was strong enough. After surgery you can become very obsessed with bodily functions and the lack of a bowel movement in four days became concerning to me. I walked and jumped up and down a little and did some deep knee bends. I peaked my head into the Chapel and wanted to go pray but tears came to my eyes just thinking about it and then I started to feel nauseated again.

I got back into bed in time for Jim and Grandma to come by after church. They walked in and said hi and I promptly threw up on Jim's shoes. What a hello! After that, the doctor, Jim and I had a little meeting. Jim could not believe that I had taken vicodin every three hours for so long. One of the things I had feared most had happened. I had a paralytic ileus, probably as a result of a combination of the anesthesia and the pain medicine.

I refused to have a nasogastric tube (a tube that was inserted through the nose into the stomach and attached to suction to empty the stomach) inserted, so my only choice was tough it out until my intestines started to move food again. The doctor ordered a suppository for me in hopes that it would help. When I vomited, I felt better briefly, but then the symptoms quickly returned. I felt like I had a rock in my stomach.

About the same time as my intestinal issues, I realized that up until the day of surgery I had been on an antidepressant medication that should not be abruptly stopped. No wonder I kept having little hallucinations like fireworks going off in my head. It was quite common for patients with a cancer diagnosis to take anti-depressant medication, as well as antianxiolytics and sleeping pills. It had now been four days without the antidepressant medication. That could account for some of my vague symptoms,

I started to sit and rock back and forth hoping to get something moving. I paced around the room. As soon as Geri got there I asked the nurses to put a sign up for all visitors to check at the desk because I did not want to see anyone else. I felt awful and was absolutely miserable and I did not want anyone to see me. I wanted off the vicodin right away since it may have been the cause of the paralytic ileus and I wanted to start on a non-narcotic pain medicine. It wasn't quite as effective but I wanted to feel better. Why any one could become addicted to vicodin was amazing to me since I felt so miserable when I took it. Believe me, there was no high. I also got a dose of the antidepressant.

You have to be so proactive when you are a patient. I kept learning this lesson over and over. There must be someone who knows every medicine that you are on and then be proactive enough to bring it up when the doctor visits. Luckily I was able to do that, but what happens when a patient can not remember or is too old?

Geri was there for the long haul. This was the hardest day for me. I was too uncomfortable to sit still so I moved around as much as possible but, I was exhausted from all the activity. We argued about which day after surgery was the worst. I said my worst day should have been yesterday but Geri said her mom thinks it was the third day after surgery which would be today. I think Geri won that argument hands down, at least her mom did. She started to look at the hundreds of catalogs my sister had left for her. We tried to laugh and joke about some of the things we saw. She was great company. I knew it was hard for her to see me so miserably uncomfortable.

I kept moving and jumping and trying to go to the bathroom. I kept taking little sips of water and took a few sips of broth for lunch. I was not going to put much in my stomach since I knew if I did, it would come right back up. I surely did not want a nasogastric tube inserted into my stomach. I was going to tough this out if it killed me.

This was the hardest thing I had been through thus far. I hurt all over and I could not take enough medicine to get pain free and I might have cancer too. It was time for me to shed more tears. I don't know where they kept coming from but the tears just kept coming. Finally about 4:00 pm I started to feel better. It had been almost 7 hours since I threw up on Jim's shoes and Geri had been with me the better part of all those hours.

I felt the mass in my stomach start to move. I was amazed to think that I could tell when my intestines were starting to function again. I felt sorry again, for my patients over the years that had experienced this discomfort. I realized the mass was probably in my intestines and not my stomach. I felt like I could stop rocking and rolling. I was able to finally go to the bathroom, the simplest of tasks. I looked at Geri and smiled because we made it. It was a small step.

Geri kept me on my toes because she wanted to know the pathophysiology of everything that had gone on or was going on. We didn't talk too much about the cancer since the pathology results would come back late tomorrow and I should go home tomorrow too. I did not feel ready to go home until now, which was late Sunday night so I was comfortable with my decision to stay one more day and leave on Monday. I was able to take a little nap and was comfortable. I finally talked Geri into going back to the house. I ate a little bit of dinner. I only felt like having soup and crackers and then some juice.

The Baseball World Series was on so I decided to watch and Jim came in about that time and was thrilled to watch the game. Maybe he was happy that I did not throw up on him again, too. We just lay together in bed and he rubbed my back. He knew how hard the day had been but needed to be home with the kids. We were just happy to be together and knew we might be dealing with heavier things later but not now. We just quietly lay together. I started to get tired about 8:30 and he left to put the kids to bed. I felt quite comfortable and knew this would be my best sleep, maybe for a long, long time.

Monday arrived with all the noise and turmoil surrounding getting discharged from the hospital. The doctor had to write the discharge orders for me to leave. Jim came early but needed to go to work so Geri would pick me up which was fine. She was off work this one last day. Another drain was discontinued and the tegaderm (see through bandage) was taken off and the dressings on my back were removed. I only needed to cover the two drain sites now. The bulky dressings on my chest had to stay for another day or two so I still looked like a DD cup. I was not ready to look at any of the operative sites on my back, so I just got dressed. Thank goodness Lisa and Nancy had given me a basket of goodies which included two shirts that zipped up the front. I could not have put anything on if it needed to go over my head. I could not move my arms and shoulders at all but I tried to get dressed by myself. I thanked the staff as I left but was a little disappointed that nursing care just was not what it used to be and they don't practice like I would want to.

Geri pulled the car around and one of the aides walked me down to the door. We sat briefly to wait and she asked me what I had been in for and I told her breast cancer and surgery. She asked if I had any risk factors and I told her no. She asked if I have taken birth control pills. I said yes, briefly, to regulate my perimenopausal cycles. She said,"Yep that'll do it." I just nodded. That'll do what, I thought to myself. I refused to feel any guilt because there are no proven links between birth control pills and breast cancer. Maybe the estrogen in the pills saved my life by enlarging the lump so I could feel it, since nothing else was abnormal. My comment was always that I was at risk because I was a woman. The day was beautiful so when Geri and I got home we sat outside for some good old sunshine. I loved the warmth of the sun. It was a shame it was so bad for us.

Chapter 7

Another Pathology Report

Grandma wanted to feed me but I was not hungry. I tried some soup and crackers which as a child I always disliked but am now thinking the dislike was overrated because it tasted really good to me right now. Grandma was trying so hard, too. I would have liked to feel celebratory but I still would not. After we ate, Geri came upstairs to keep me company while I napped. I was tired and hurting and needed to lie down. I kept telling her she needed to go back home to get ready to go back to work. She was not going to budge because the pathology report was due back any moment.

I got a little sleep and I was so cold. My feet were like ice cubes. Geri rubbed my feet until they got warm. Thank you God for taking care of me, I thought. Neighbors brought a meal that night. I was actually downstairs briefly, talked to them and thanked them. They did not stay long at all. Starting today dinner would come every Monday and Wednesday and I had a cook who came on Thursdays and made two dinners for the week, so we were well taken care of. Neither Grandma nor anyone else had to worry about meals.

My anxiety level elevated as we kept vigil by the phone. Finally when it was time to eat dinner, I realized that we would not get any information today. I was so disconcerted and I was weepy again because I knew Geri had to leave and I had wanted her with me when I received the report. There was just no telling when we would get any information, now. It was a very subdued dinner. We were all so disappointed but no one really wanted to admit to that, because they did not want me to get upset. Maybe no news was good news or maybe not. I was thrilled to be home with the kids but could not give them a big hug because of the pain all over my body. After dinner Geri took off, very disappointed that we had not received any news. I was sad to see her go but knew she needed to go to work and who knew when I might need her to come back. Grandma was only able to stay another few days because she had health issues she needed to take care of at home.

I wanted to take another shower and Jim had to help this time. This became quite a production again. I told him about the garbage bags to keep all my incisions dry. He looked at me like I had lost my mind but was very helpful. I did look pretty funny, again. He decided the easiest thing was to take a shower with me. This seemed a bit excessive. He finished up with his shower and then I got in. It was pretty crowded in the shower and under other circumstances this would be fairly romantic. He shampooed my hair and about shook my head off in doing so. I finished in the bath since I did not have a hand held shower head. Once again all the incisions stayed dry and now all we had to do was change the dressings on the drains. One was leaking a lot, around the drain, but the other was still draining into the drain. I was going to see the plastic surgeon in two days so we reinforced the dressing fairly often.

We were so disappointed not to have heard about the pathology report we just could not speak about it. We just went to bed without any discussion. Getting into bed was a hassle and required a lot of time to get propped up on pillows and to get comfortable. Before going to bed, I decided to brush my teeth. That in and of itself was not a major milestone, but for some reason tonight when I brushed my teeth it was with a little more vigor than in the hospital and as I brushed, my breasts moved up and down. This was a very weird sensation and I thought it was totally bizarre until I realized that the latissimus dorsi muscle was still doing what it was supposed to do even though it had been moved. It was still trying to help move my shoulder up and down, even though it was not where it should have been. Every time I brushed my teeth or combed my hair, the latissimus would be innervated and strange movements would happen. I remembered that it would take a few months for the muscle to quit acting like it was supposed to and I had to adjust to the breasts moving up and down. Another addition to my list, *things your doctor never tells you.*

Tonight I took my normal tranquilizer and sleeping pills as well as pain medicine. I really needed to sleep given what was to come tomorrow. I awakened during the night to take pain medicine and was up the next morning in time to see the kids off to school. This was important to maintain a routine that was normal since I did not want them to think I was sick. That day I started to see the bus off, wave, and blow a kiss every day. I vowed to keep it up for fear I might not be around to do it very much longer. I have continued it to this very day. I immediately laid down on the couch to rest.

I could not bear to get into bed, since it required such effort to get comfortable, but I needed to rest. I tried to relax by meditating using a mantra but that was a lost cause so I just closed my eyes and prayed. This was the beginning of what I liked to call my Jesus meditation. Pretty soon I dozed a bit. I was still very much on edge because surely the pathology report would come back today. I expected that I might not get word until late in the day.

Well, Jim must have gotten impatient, because he called at 10:30 am. He had called the pathologist himself and gotten the results. Oh my gosh, how could he do that? Being an insider helped a lot. This was all backward. My doctor was the one who should have called me. The news was not good and not at all what we expected. They had found two other tumors of the left breast. One was bigger than the original tumor. This one was 2.1 cm. Furthermore of the 22 lymph nodes taken, one was positive for micro-metastatic disease. How could this be? Everyone said there was nothing to worry about and the cancer would be gone. It could have been worse. I could have had multiple lymph nodes positive, instead of just one. The exact diagnosis was a breast carcinoma, infiltrating ductal type slightly larger than 2 cm. (capable of and was spreading to the surrounding breast) They also found a ductal carcinoma in situ (totally located in one spot and not spreading) with a minor component of

121

neoplasm. They also found evidence of fibrocystic disease (lumpy breasts) which was no big deal but why in the world did I not know about it? Then there was the lymph node. Micrometastatic disease, I later found out, is almost like no disease. I knew, however, that result would push me into chemotherapy. This was an answer to my prayer that if I required chemotherapy that just one lymph node be positive. It was a strange prayer request. How would I tell everyone this news? My inner circle had felt so optimistic. My ten year survival dropped from 90% to 70% in about a minute and a half. I plugged the new information into the Mayo Clinic website right away. How could I get through this huge setback? What in the world would I do now? How could I face this after everything else I had been through? How could I put my family through more and how would my father cope? So many questions. My optimism went out the window. This day had been a circus and it was only beginning. Needless to say, I cried all day. Thankfully Jim's mom was still here but she cried too. I called my dad and told him I had good and bad news. He wanted to know what the good news was. I said I guess there wasn't any but the report could have been worse. He did not see anything positive at all and could not imagine how the news could have been worse.

Jim talked to the oncologist and got an appointment for that afternoon at 4:30. It was wonderful to get in so quickly, but I was not sure I was ready to drive into Boulder and put on a brave front. It was snowing and gray and blustery outside. It suited our moods. Finally I got phone calls from the oncologist and the surgeon. The surgeon apologized profusely for not calling me the day before just to tell me she had heard nothing.

I don't remember the trip into Boulder at all. I was in my own little world, probably of self pity. Predictably, we went through the weight taking just like the first visit. Then we were put in a room. First the oncologist said, "I have good news, you don't need radiation." I was not sure if that was good or not. I was not too sure of anything at that moment except that I was an emotional wreck. Then he apologized for being so wrong and acknowledged that I had certainly chosen the right option for my surgery. I made sure I told him to never underestimate the sixth sense of a nurse. We knew the right thing to do most of the time and I knew my body really well. I did feel betrayed by my body, by life, by medicine, and by God. I started to pray a lot about that. I knew, deep down, that God would never betray me.

The oncologist started presenting Jim and me with all of the options for treatment and my mind raced. With the oncologist was a clinical nurse researcher and she started to explain the different clinical trials that might be of interest to me. I could be in a clinical trial but I would not necessarily know if I was getting trial medicine or regular medicine. I could receive standard treatment which would be four sessions of chemotherapy with Doxorubicin and Cyclophosamide. This was the gold standard of breast cancer chemotherapy. These have been used for years so I was familiar with both. There would be four sessions three weeks apart. I knew about the six course treatment so four was better or at least I thought so. I would go through menopause, feel miserable, have no libido, feel tired and then be on tamoxifen for five years. It had a lot of side effects but we would deal with all of that later. This sounded like a life sentence in solitary confinement with no chance for parole. Breast cancer had already consumed my life for six weeks and it appeared it would consume my life forever. I wondered if a cancer victim ever got over the panic.

We discussed all the statistics and percentages for survival with all the different medications. None sounded good. Basically I had a 70% chance of being alive in ten years. I wanted to know the bottom line. What if I did absolutely nothing? What were my chances then? There was a 50% chance of being alive in ten years. What happened to five year survival? I understood that they used ten years now because if you lived that long you were considered cured at that point. When I was in nursing school, we were concerned about the five year survival. Tomorrow seemed a long way off, much less ten years. If only I were 65 instead of 47? This would be far easier to take although I'm not sure why. I had young children. The boys would remember me but what about Kate? I waited so long to have this little girl, how could I leave her and have her not remember me? I started to think of all the graduations and weddings and grandchildren I would miss. I tried to pay attention to what the doctor was saying to me, but my mind kept wandering. I was only 5 days out from surgery and I had a fair amount of medication in my system. Everything hurt and I was nauseous. That was beginning to feel like the only thing that I could count on anymore.

The thoughts in my head were spinning out of control, which was just as my life was spinning out of control as well. Armed with all the information and lots of paperwork we left for home. It was snowing and for some reason unknown to anyone, Boulder had the worst traffic jam in years. I sobbed quietly or sat staring out the window. It was wet and miserable and exactly mimicked how I felt. What must Jim be thinking? We can't even bring ourselves to talk. I had five hot flashes in the next half hour. Maybe I'm already menopausal. I had never wished for something so silly but it would be better for my survival if I were postmenopausal. It had taken us almost an hour to go a few miles. The traffic was not moving at all so we tried another route. Same thing; dead stop. There must be an accident somewhere because we saw only thousands of tail lights and head lights. Could this day have gotten any worse? I wanted a glass of wine. I was still crying and now I had to go to the bathroom and there was nowhere to stop. I was so thirsty but I had finished all my water taking my last pain medication in the car. The car had as much water and snow on it as I seemed to be crying. I sure had a lot of tears. We saw a *Wendy's* and decided to stop and go to the bathroom. The restaurant was packed with annoyed commuters who clearly had come in from the cold with the intention of waiting it out. They all seemed to be in this restaurant. We made it to the bathroom and back to the car. The traffic was still as bad and just getting out of the parking lot took a fair amount of skill. The roads were not slick at all but the people driving were very impatient and we were only moving at a snail's pace. It was painfully slow.

Was it only this morning that I found out that I had cancer, again? Finally on our way again I made one decision and shared it with Jim. I was not going to go into a clinical trial. That would extend my treatment by two months and cause many more side effects. My body was just not strong enough for that right now and I was not strong enough to deal with that either. Jim was in agreement with anything I said at this point. What if I had gone in for only a lumpectomy thinking radiation would be all I needed. I'd be facing another surgery or maybe not. I might not have known that the second tumor was even there. I might have been dead within a few years. I had more than a few people think I was overcalling on the surgery option. At least I did not need another surgery. Who cared about nipples? I did not need them and I did not want any more surgery.

How were we going to face the kids and the phone calls we needed to make when we arrived home? Jerred my oldest son was in college in California and was under the impression that things were fine and everything looked benign. How could I tell him any of this when he was trying to concentrate on his studies? I really wanted to hide away by myself with my head in the sand somewhere and wish this whole ordeal away. I still just could not accept that this actually happened to me. These things always happened to other people.

Prayer was always good for me but how and what would I pray for now? I wanted to be cured but that cannot happen or if it did, it would take years before I was certain of anything. Even then, there was no certainty. This cancer could recur anywhere at anytime. I found myself asking God what it was that I needed.

I sure did not know. I knew God would provide an answer because that is what faith was based on, but I just could not imagine how he would answer my prayers.

Earlier in the day the insurance company had called and insisted that I see a psychiatrist. Why in the world did I need to see a psychiatrist? I had a fatal disease and a psychiatrist could not cure it. This was a hurdle I could deal with later. I did not have the time or the inclination to research psychiatrists. I was impressed that the insurance company was so aware of what was going on. A nurse, who was a breast cancer consultant for the insurance company, telephoned the day I found out I had breast cancer again. The nurse wanted me to schedule an appointment with the psychiatrist. Though the timing was difficult and I cried through the phone call, seeing a shrink was the last thing on my mind. I started to think about hair loss and other side effects of chemotherapy and I became totally overwhelmed. You really needed to take this all in small doses. The traffic started to clear by the time we got to Louisville near our home.

Two hours and ten minutes later and many phone calls to Grandma, we finally pulled into the garage at 8:30 pm. I could not face the kids, but dinner was ready and we tried to choke some down. The rest of the family, thankfully, had eaten hours ago. I had to make a few phone calls, one to Janet and one to Nancy. I had already called Geri in the middle of a class because she wanted to know immediately after I found out the pathology results and she had left her phone on all day. She was not concentrating very well on her classes. Bad or good, she was emphatic that she be informed immediately. While I was on the phone, Jim told the kids the latest news. I was trying to get up enough courage to tell the kids when I found out that he had already done so. I thought I would have liked to have been with him but what was done was done. I would have cried anyway. I could not bear to tell Jerred yet. Sometime during the evening Jim went across the street and talked to Nancy. She gave him a big hug and cried and asked him why God had not answered all of our prayers and how this could have happened? How could everyone have been so optimistic only to have this happen? So many people were praying for the outcome to be good. Why did God not answer our prayers? I felt a lot helpless and a little hopeless right now. I tried to relax as I fell asleep and prayed for God's guidance.

As I lay awake early the next morning I started to feel a little empowered, but only just a little. My sleeping pills were great but only lasted about five hours so it was about five in the morning when I awakened. Jim was not awake yet but I came to the realization that I could choose to do nothing at all and I still had a 50/50 chance of ten year survival. That was not all that bad and it would be my decision if I made it. I would be in control. I felt a bit stronger. I did not have to feel guilty about not doing a clinical trial. Even though I was a nurse and felt research was critical. I did not have to choose to be in a clinical trial. A little more empowerment. This whole situation was torture but I felt a tremendous relief to be in some control. *Yes God, I was listening.* I told Jim the minute he awakened and maybe I even woke him up a little early. I was so excited I wanted to share it. He was not quite as excited about my revelation as I was, but, was happy I felt some control.

It was October 30th and thankfully Grandma was here and doing a great job with the kids. She did not need to worry about much cooking since my neighbors had really taken that over so she only had to keep up with the laundry and the kids. I certainly did not want her to get sick. Thank goodness she was here because I was not as likely to sit and brood as I would have had I been alone. In 77 years she had never had the ability to just leave home for a lengthy period of time with so little notice. To have that ability when we needed her most was something of a miracle and certainly an answer to prayer.

I was obsessing about my breasts. They were too big and got in my way. Maybe I should not have had the reconstructive surgery. They even made my back hurt because I thought they pulled me over with their weight. I was scheduled to see the plastic surgeon the following day so I would see what she said. I was still bandaged on my chest so that did make me seem terribly buxom. Whatever was I thinking when I decided to get the reconstruction done? I might not even live to enjoy the boobs. My recovery was certainly longer because of the major surgery involved. A simple mastectomy would have meant I was in and out the same day. Recovery from major surgery was a six week ordeal.

I decided I needed to schedule two naps into my day and during that time I would meditate and visualize. Twice a day seemed good right now since it would give me something to concentrate on besides my life unfolding in front of me. I wanted to take good care of myself and get into some good habits before Grandma left. I started a bit hesitantly but I felt more relaxed as I finished each rest period. As I rested I tried to visualize my cancer and plan the attack with my White Blood Cells. I was not crazy about the war model but it was a place to start. I formulated something less violent. I still cried all the time. Every time I opened my mouth to say anything my eyes welled up with tears.

I had an appointment with the plastic surgeon today and Jim was able to go with me. I mustered up the energy and tried to hold back the tears before we left. The office was subdued when we got there. It was still very peaceful with the waterfall but my previous excitement seemed to be muted. The plastic surgeon was so excited, she was animated. She said as soon as she got the pathology report she called the surgeon and the oncologist to make sure that I would not need radiation. Radiation and implants were a horrible combination. Radiation destroyed the implants by hardening them and the skin around the radiation site. She was like a little kid in the candy store when she told me that it was great not to get radiation. I tried to be excited but tears choked me. When she took off the bandages she was ecstatic. My breasts looked just awesome to her. I mentioned that they might be too big. She looked a bit disheartened. "Don't you like them?" she asked. Well yes of course I did, but this whole thing was just too much. I still had tape everywhere and a drain in and where the tape had come off my skin was burned and bright red. I guessed I was having a little trouble seeing the big picture because of all the little minor annoyances. Now I hoped all the bandages would be gone.

I had to keep my left breast bound very tightly on the lateral side so that the implant would not slide under my arm. There's something I never saw coming. With all the work done to my left breast and with the lymph node dissection, there was nothing to hold the implant in place except the doctor had sutured my donor muscle to my intercostal muscle between my ribs to keep the implant in place. If she hadn't done this I might have ended up with the implant in my armpit. That's not a nice picture in my mind! No wonder I could barely move my arm! I had stitches everywhere. I also had this very strange fibrous, tendon in the middle of my armpit that made it look as if I had two armpits on the left side. It was very tight and made it hard to move my arms but that was hard anyway because it hurt. She gave me a few ideas for the massive amount of tape that I must use, because she saw how badly my skin had reacted to the previous tape. She taped the left breast up again. I needed to continue doing this for another six weeks. But, oh by the way, if you wedged a sanitary pad into your bra, that would keep the shape too. That was the first sensible thing I had heard in a long time. So far I had no bra which I could comfortably wear since I now needed an extra large size to get around me, the tape, and the sanitary napkin. I could take a shower now without the garbage bag. This was success, in a world where I had limited capabilities. I was ready to get back on my feet and I was depressed that I was not progressing faster. After all I was 6 days out from surgery. I should be back running miles by now. I guess I was not too realistic. I asked if I could start to exercise. The doctor thought about that one for awhile and her answer was yes as long as I did not use my arms. I can slowly start back on my elliptical trainer without the arms. Exercise was a tremendous stress reliever for me. I wanted to do this.

Sleeping was just about the most difficult thing to do right then. I had to lie on my back and since I was a stomach person, it was virtually impossible to change. But, everything was possible when necessity dictated. The plastic surgeon wanted no pressure on the new breasts for six weeks. That ruled out sleeping on my stomach if I could even have gotten there. I was in a fair amount of pain and now I worried about the cancer and the need for chemotherapy.

I awakened a lot between the pain from the surgery and the anxiety associated with the cancer diagnosis. When I lay there alone I was so scared. Jim's snoring became worse over the years. I thought it ran in his family. They all snored loud enough to wake the dead. Strangely enough right now, I found that his snoring was unbelievably reassuring. When I awakened at night and couldn't sleep, if I heard the snoring, I knew that I was not alone and I was alive. I even told Jim that his snoring provided me peace. Neither of us could believe it. I would never complain about it again because I felt so blessed to have him there beside me. God was watching out for me and changing my behaviors. I did not even know what to pray for sometimes but He knew.

It was Halloween, and my least favorite day of the year. I disliked it now and always had, except when I was little. I loved to dress up and get candy. Now, it made me nauseous. Kate was swinging off of chandeliers, she was so excited. She was a princess for at least the third year in a row. Thank goodness I could still convince her it was a great costume. She'll grow out of it this year though. I trudged through the day with no particular thoughts or revelations.

I should call to make an appointment with the psychiatrist because the insurance company wanted me to call back with dates and times. They were going to force this issue. I didn't think I could complete a thought much less delve into anything else the psychiatrist might find. My mind was fuzzy from the anesthesia and pretty soon it would be fuzzy from the chemotherapy. It was a lose-lose situation. I tried to engage Jim in conversation about our lives and where we would go from here. I was afraid he would go looking for a new partner since this one was so scarred up and nonfunctional now. Of course I ended up in tears again. He did not want to even think about this. Trick or treat was finally over. It was freezing cold and not too many kids were braving the weather. Every time the door opened I just shivered as the draft rushed in. My hands and feet were so cold that I did not think they would ever warm up again. The weather was gray and snowy, so it went along with my feelings and my very cold hands and feet.

The days seemed to all blur together. I kept trying to make all these plans but I was just a robot on a roller coaster and did not know whether I should laugh or cry.

I did not know if this was a blessing or a curse. I liked everyone home with me but the days just lingered. When Monday came I got depressed all over again. I now found out that I had even more people around the country praying for me. Through family and friends I was on many prayer chains in churches and schools. I found tremendous strength and comfort in that. I felt the peace that I wanted to feel as a result of those prayers. Otherwise, I was only at peace when I slept; as soon as I awakened I was in a panic as I waited for something bad to happen. I think back on the words from the song Jesus

Loves Me. "Jesus loves me this I know, for the Bible tells me so." It was the first song I learned in Sunday school. That gave me peace.

Grandma had to leave in a few days, quite reluctantly too. She was so worried about how I would do with chemotherapy, which started in less than two weeks. We were all a bit anxious about that. Geri would be here the day Grandma left so I would have company and support. I can't imagine what I would do without her and yet this must disrupt her life a lot. I felt like I was dying a little bit every day. The kids just went along as usual. Kate had a dance recital but I could not go. Jim needed to go. I did not want to be out in public. I was certain I had a big C tattooed on my head for cancer and everyone felt sorry for me. My friends and neighbors kept me amazed with their outpouring of food and love. So many things we don't appreciate until we faced immense hardship. The cards and uplifting scripture verses kept appearing in my special box. I checked it many times a day.

One day as I lay on the couch meditating and praying, my mother-in-law was next to me on the other couch. I cried again because those tears were uncontrollable. As I lay there I heard a voice tell me I was not going to die. I could not tell where the voice was coming from but it was very reassuring. I felt my anxiety begin to drain out of me and be replaced by a golden warmth. The warmth seemed to come from over my shoulder. I tried to make it come back but I couldn't. I decided my mind must be playing some kind of a trick on me, or maybe it was just wishful thinking. When I told Janet about this she decided it was our mom with a glass of ginger ale. When we were sick as kids, mom would bring us ginger ale and we were sure to feel better. I think it was God trying to tell me I was just fine and not to worry. I believed that God talked to me in that moment.

As October drew to a close, Breast Cancer Awareness month would soon be over. I had been inundated with information, both good and bad. I resolved to make women more proactive when it came to breast cancer awareness and I wanted to run the Race for the Cure next year. It meant a lot to me and I wanted my whole family to participate. This disease was curable and I intended to be a part of the cure. I finally told Jerred about the cancer. He seemed so far away in California, at school, but we really could not put off telling him any more. Jennie, his girlfriend's mother had been through many lumpectomies and chemotherapy and she was a twelve year survivor. I needed someone to talk to who had been through this. I momentarily thought a support group would be a terrific idea. Later I researched on the Internet to find one and could not seem to find a good fit.

Jerred was stunned and wanted to know how this could be since every doctor said it looked like nothing. Life happened. I did not know how everyone could be so wrong, but they were and now we had to deal with it. Jerred would be home in three weeks for Thanksgiving, which I thought would be good because he'd realize that we were going on with our activities and life as normal as possible. That was, everyone but me. I tried to take really good care of myself and stay healthy as I prepared to receive the chemotherapy which I absolutely did not want.

Prior to my surgery I had resolved to make dietary changes following the surgery. I was going to cut out all caffeine. I did not drink a lot of coffee, but I did like it in the morning. I never had any more caffeine after the surgery and if I had withdrawal headaches, I didn't know it, since I was so miserable with all the other post surgery problems. I planned that well. I also decided to decrease fat from our diets and include more fish and vegetarian meals. I didn't know if this would be helpful but at least I felt in control of this aspect of our lives. I was also going to increase my fruit and vegetable intake to six to nine servings a day instead of five. Additionally I would try to eliminate refined sugar as well as increasing complex carbohydrates. My family would derive benefits from this diet but they would not realize it for years. I did not actually believe in diets. I think healthy is a balance between the intake of good, healthy food and getting enough exercise. I certainly did not advocate anything more than common sense and moderation.

The estate portfolio manager for my dad's estate arrived for a visit. It had been three very long months since my mom died and we had quite a few questions. Luckily my brother Harvey was here, but they wanted me to be present at the meetings as well. I felt like I should be dealing with my own estate plans. I was afraid I was closer to dying than my dad... I tried to keep those thoughts to myself, despite thinking this meeting was totally unnecessary for me to attend unless it was to discuss plans for my own estate.

My surgical scars began to heal but my breasts still felt too big. The implants seemed to slosh a bit, too. I had finally gotten creative with the taping of my left breast. I found an extra large sport bra that I stuck a sanitary pad in for support and then taped the lateral side of my breast so that the least amount of tape touched my skin as was possible. I was proud of myself for figuring this out since the original tape burns were still painful and that discomfort made me not want to do what I needed to do to support the left breast. I must say the shape of my left breast was quite nice. Earlier in my post operative period, I thought the right breast looked better, because my arm did not rub against it, but actually the shape was not nearly as natural as the left. It was also already starting to form a scar capsule and that was not particularly good. It was inevitable because when a foreign object, like an implant was put in your body, the body tried to separate it from the rest of the body, by forming a scar around it. The only action I could take proactively was to massage both breasts every day with lotion or massage oil and try to keep the scar capsule formation to a minimal. Since this was a continual process, 1 was not sure that I would ever be able to stop the massage. Here was another area where health care could be a bit more progressive. I was learning how to do this all on my own but someone should be able to incorporate it into massage therapy or even physical therapy. It would certainly benefit everyone with an implant to at least learn the correct technique for this type of massage.

Kate had dance class and I needed to take her since no one else was home. I did not want to go out, but I got my stiff upper lip and managed to get her to class and tell the teacher that I would be undergoing chemotherapy. She was stunned too, since like everyone else she thought the prognosis was better than that. She asked if she could share the information with the other parents since they were beginning to sense that something was wrong. One parent already knew so I told her that was fine. There were very few secrets in a small town. I really didn't intend for this to be a secret either because I wanted to educate as long as I was going through this. The registered nurse part of me still wanted to educate as many people as I could to never stop doing breast self exams, getting yearly mammograms, and seeing one's physician for a thorough exam every year. The woman side of me still wanted to stick my head in the sand and wish this away. I started this ordeal proactively and that is how I intended to continue.

The Cancer Center contacted me to see if I was getting in all the appointments I needed. Of course not, I was just sitting around trying to figure out what came next. I was also trying to recover from major surgery and the diagnosis of cancer. That seemed like enough, but in order to start chemotherapy, I needed to get a MUGA Heart Scan. The scan would give the oncologist information on how well my heart was pumping blood. I would have dye injected into a vein and the scan would look at the function of the left side of my heart. Yet more information I had to assimilate. The doxorubicin (one of my chemotherapy agents) was heart toxic and could cause heart failure and eventually the need for a heart transplant. It was very rare but baseline information was needed before they could proceed with the treatments. A heart transplant! I just did not know what else I could deal with. I must have a very healthy heart since I have been an athlete since junior high school. I just knew that exercise would pay off somewhere down the road. It had to.

I also needed to schedule having a port inserted for chemotherapy to be given. This was news to me. I had no idea they would not just start an intravenous line every time I had a treatment. Oh no, the port was much easier. It was a semi permanent vessel that allowed access to a major vein for the duration of treatment. It however required going back into the operating room and same day surgery and more medicine for conscious sedation. Not another surgery! I was still recovering from the previous surgeries. I think that it's time now to get my head out of the sand. The sooner we started, the sooner we finished. Although with breast cancer, nothing was ever finished.

There really was no good way to follow breast cancer patients after treatment. There's no blood test or tumor marker. According to my oncologist, it sounded like you flew by the seat of your pants. You never really knew the status of the cancer. I needed to get some perspective and a coping mechanism in place. I was not used to such uncertainty. I was falling apart and had no precedents to bring into play to help me cope now.

When all else eluded me, I started to exercise more. I was very weak and started on the elliptical trainer for just a few minutes a day. I also tried to get 20 minutes of sunshine everyday if the sun was out. Sometimes I lay down on the floor in my bedroom with the door to the deck open and sometimes I sat on the front porch. I wanted to get some direct sun so my pineal gland would produce melatonin and I would sleep at night. I still had hair so no one knew what was really up. Within a few days I got the MUGA scan of the heart. Everything scared me to death now. What if I reacted to the radioactive contrast they had to inject? What if I had some existing heart problem that we never knew about? I had a sister who died of Tetralogy of Fallot when she was a few days old. That was a congenital abnormality that (at that time) was a fatal trans- positioning of the major arteries leaving the heart. A heart problem was not that far fetched since we already had one in the family. I had an active imagination and it was working overtime. I was athletic and a 21 year veteran of the army. I would have dropped dead years ago with something serious if there were anything wrong with my heart.

With a little more time on my hands I still tried to do Christian meditation twice a day and prayed as often as possible. After taking my cleansing breaths, I focused on small bits of scripture, or the Lord's Prayer, or I just said Jesus over and over to get to that relaxed point. Amazingly it worked and it did not take me long before I had mastered the skill. I called it my Jesus meditation. I liked it and looked forward to it every day. I continued with my visualization too. I had finally decided to view my White Blood Cells as huge puffy stars that filled all the blood vessels in my body and as the stars moved along they wiped out the bad cancer cells like one would wipe off a dry erase board. There was no residual after the white board was clean. I had experimented with other visuals but I liked this nonviolent, clean one. Chalk boards create dust, but dry erase boards were clean.

I still awakened in the middle of the night near panic and sometimes during the day I became paralyzed with anxiety. What if I died? What would my kids do? How could medical science have let me down so much? I knew people kept me in their prayers but maybe I needed to pray for myself. Before the anxiety got bad I started to pray immediately that it would go away. I prayed short, direct little prayers and I was overcome with peace. Then I asked God to keep me at peace. When I prayed, the gnawing pit in my stomach went away. I needed to learn to give up my burdens and live. During these few days I had also formulated a plan for keeping myself busy. I was behind on my kid's scrapbooks as well as one I was working on for Jim and me. There were easily three or four months of work just to catch up to the present. Poor Jerred was supposed to get his finished scrapbook for graduation from High School eighteen months ago but I had never gotten it finished. I was determined to be productive during chemotherapy when I believed I needed to stay in the house and away from harmful germs.

I finally got the courage to go and see the psychiatrist. Of course I burst into tears before I walked into her office. I assured her that I was really fine, but she had a series of questions for me. She wanted to know if I was suicidal which made sense. Of course, I was not. She was as puzzled as I was why the insurance company wanted this encounter. I hated seeing a psychiatrist and I hated answering all the questions. Before I left, she assured me that all my tears were perfectly normal given everything I had been through, but just to be on the safe side she wanted to see me one more time before Christmas.

Chapter 8

Chemotherapy

On Friday, November 8th, four days before chemotherapy, the Cancer Center called again. This time they told me I needed to come in to sign all my consent forms and get pre-chemotherapy counseling. Another thing I either chose not to remember or was never told about. I was not getting the memos about what I was supposed to be getting done. It seemed to me that someone should be responsible for telling me about these things to help me get through the puzzle. The Cancer Center had an opening this afternoon. I had not driven at all since surgery and I was petrified to drive that far but I had no choice. No one could drive me so I was off to the appointment. I felt better driving than I thought I would. I was extremely careful though because I could not turn around to look out all the windows as well as usual. My head, neck, shoulders and chest were still pretty tight and sore.

I arrived and was called back right away. Those nurses were always on time. I expected to not like the nurse based on the information she would have to give me. There was no rationale but I just thought this was going to be a horrible experience. She was quite the opposite. She was very calm and likeable and, I thought, very competent. She was an oncology nurse and had special training, and she had done this for years and still loved it. I wondered how she could surround herself with death all the time. First she went over the risks and hazards of treatment. This included a list about a mile long of every awful thing that you could imagine, except getting hit by a truck. The highlights were lung damage, kidney damage, heart damage, and hearing loss. Lesser problems were anemia, low white blood cell count, and mouth sores. Then in bold letters the form read: **Do not sign this unless you thoroughly understand this**. I understood but not thoroughly since I still did not understand why I was the one here. That's the woman in me again getting a bit histrionic. The nurse in me knew they were required to give me all this information. Those of us in health care call it informed consent. I signed the form and we moved on to the next form. This was a patient teaching form. This detailed exactly what medicine I would get and all the adverse reactions that I needed to report to the oncologist's office. I wanted to know just how bad this would be. No one seemed to be able to answer that, or more probable, they did not want to answer because it was so awful. I expected the absolute worst but the nurse told me that it varied dramatically from patient to patient. She also told me to avoid crowds and churches and schools since these places are all germ laden. I would be immunosuppressed and unable to fight off common illnesses. Wow, I took care of people like that but I never expected to be one! Thankfully I had gotten my flu shot about a week before surgery. I was given a handout on everything I should be doing and shouldn't be doing. It was about 20 pages long. I could read that when I got home along with the specific side effects of each of the chemotherapeutic agents I would be getting. None of this information was good. Everything seemed like an adverse effect. She also gave me all the prescriptions for the anti-nausea medications to fill today since I might like to do that before the day of chemotherapy.

This was also my first opportunity to see the area where they administered the chemotherapy. It was freezing and very scary looking. There was a lot of equipment and computers and chairs and rooms with beds. The area where the nurses prepared the chemotherapy looked like the inside of a spaceship. The measurement of the amount of chemotherapy was extremely precise and thus necessitated the computers and exact dosage preparation equipment. Chemotherapy was 'chemical treatment', just like the word sounds, that involved giving near toxic amounts of different drugs depending on the type of cancer. Although new drug regimens were being researched, I would be getting the gold standard of treatment for breast cancer, which had been around for many years. Unfortunately it was controlled poisoning. The drugs killed rapidly replicating cells, cancer cells as well as other cells within the body that are similar, like hair follicle cells, skin cells, and mucosal cells like those of the mouth and intestinal system, and most importantly some white blood cells, which were responsible for the immune system. Sometimes so many white blood cells were lost that a bone marrow transplant became necessary to give the body back the ability to form the white blood cells.

The big room had a lot of chairs that looked like recliners. I can't imagine just sitting around with a room full of people I don't know receiving controlled poisoning. I liked the private room with two recliners and the TV/VCR. I never go to movies, but typically wait to see them when they come out on video. If laughter was the best medicine, a comedy might be good during the treatments. I finally left after about an hour. It was a lot to take in all at once but I was getting used to the regular sessions of information overload. It was so overwhelming but I was going on this adventure whether I wanted to or not. It helped me to look at it as an adventure which gave the journey a little excitement, kind of like going on a very exotic vacation or a dangerous mission. The problem was that this journey would last the rest of my life, and whether that would be ten or twenty or more years, I had no way of knowing. This was surely a better approach than some other ways I could imagine. I bought everything that was suggested to prevent some side effects, like soft bristle toothbrushes so my gums wouldn't bleed and easy to digest foods to eat if I felt nauseous, the mere mention of it made me want to wretch. I filled the prescriptions for anticoagulants and antiemetics and was on my way home. And of course, I went home and read everything that I received cover to cover.

My port (the means by which the medicine would be administered to me intravenously) was placed on Monday, Veteran's Day. That was hardly the way I wanted to celebrate as a veteran. I was little nervous about this procedure too. I planned this procedure at a different hospital which was further away, but I got the appointment earlier. This was the hospital where my general surgeon usually worked. There was not a crowd. It was very peaceful and although I had to wait quite awhile to get called, it was a nice chance to talk to Jim. That gnawing pit was in my stomach again. I had to explain to everyone what was going on and they all knew I had breast cancer. I still can't get used to the diagnosis much less say it. As soon as I received conscious sedation, I felt better. Conscious sedation made me feel relaxed and coupled with pain medication allowed simple procedures to be accomplished without general anesthesia. I was becoming a professional at getting this powerful medicine. I was awake as the port was placed, and I had a shooting pain into my shoulder blade when the surgeon injected the area above my right collar bone with the numbing medicines, marcaine and xylocaine. Apparently that happened to some people, and I was one of the lucky few. My surgeon did not really know why, but it was excruciating and unrelenting. As she inserted the catheter into my subclavian vein I asked how it won't come loose and become a huge floating embolus (clot) through my heart and into my lungs that would kill me. Well that could happen but she would secure the catheter really well to the port itself which was about the size of a quarter. I felt the catheter being inserted and I suddenly started to experience ectopic or abnormal extra heart beats. Those were beats that originated in a different area of the heart and followed a different pathway through the heart than a regular heart beat. I calmly asked why I was having the ectopic beats and whether they would be permanent. I knew that when a catheter was inserted into the right atrium of the heart it would cause these ectopic beats. I remembered that from years working in the ICU. The surgeon assured me that they only did that to make sure they were in the right atrium and she pulled the catheter back so it sat just outside the heart in the vena cava. From here, no unusual heartbeats would be initiated. That was fine by me. Then she attached the port and sewed the catheter securely in place. I felt the tugging as she did this. I was not in pain but I did feel pressure and movement. I'm sure she put in an extra suture just so I would not worry about the catheter coming loose.

Within an hour the catheter was in place and I was out of the operating room. Since chemotherapy started tomorrow, November 12th, she had inserted a needle and tubing into the port while the area was numb so the nurses would not have to stick me in the morning since the site would be very tender. Then the surgeon also filled the port and tubing with heparin, a medicine that would keep the port from clotting off and becoming useless. The surgeon asked if I wanted any medication for pain. Not a chance. I would be fine with something non-narcotic and I had some left from surgery. Now I also must go on a very small dose of coumadin to prevent clotting of the port and catheter until they pulled it out. Coumadin is better known as the main ingredient in rat poison and is also the medicine that contributed to my mother's death just a few months earlier. How reassuring that all was. It seemed like years before this port would come out. It will actually be next year, 2003. It was very uncomfortable on the ride home because the seatbelt rubbed right on top of the bandaged port. I had drawn my bra line on my chest and tried to help with the port's placement. I guess I could not avoid the seatbelt though, unless I was the driver instead of on the passenger's side, or just stayed home. The next morning was the beginning of chemotherapy. I struggled to eat something since from all the horror stories I have heard, I might not eat for another week. I cannot be certain I slept that night at all. I dreaded the chemotherapy but I would be 25% done with the treatments at the end of the day. My prayers to God to keep my anxiety away were working. That's called answered prayer. The next morning we got the kids off to school and prepared to leave. Jim was going to take me to my first treatment. I had all the rest of the treatments planned out and marked on my calendar so I would be done around the 12th of January. That's a long way off but I could do this.

The drive in to Boulder was becoming very familiar and it always felt a bit like I was going to the guillotine. I was already nauseous and I hadn't even gotten any medication yet. When we arrived, I signed in and got blood drawn and had my weight taken and sat in a room to see the doctor before the chemotherapy. This was a routine I would become very familiar with over the next few months. Today the oncologist recalculated my doses of chemotherapy and showed them to me so I knew them as well. This was, after all, a very refined method of controlled poisoning. You could not be too careful and I liked the control of knowing my dosages. I must have seemed quite anxious, crying several times during my exam because he ordered a dose of lorazepam (antianxiety medication) to calm me down prior to treatment. I was still praying and hanging in there, but I was still frightened.

First they checked to make sure that the port was open and then started with a dose of steroid in the IV. The nurse warned me that the steroid would keep me awake all that night unless I took a sleeping medication. Then I received antinausea medication, the one my insurance company authorized. The insurance company always seemed to get the last word. Then the moment of truth, the doxorubicin arrived. The syringe was huge and it was the most frightening looking medicine because it was red! The red bullet. I now understand that nickname. My eyes were as big as saucers, but the oncology nurse was the same one who had done my counseling a few days earlier so I felt very comfortable with her. The doxorubicin was given IV push with a large syringe (rather than over time in a bag) by the nurse because throughout the dosing, they checked whether or not the catheter was in the correct location since the medication was so toxic. If it got outside of the vein it caused such bad necrosis (tissue death), that people needed skin grafts to repair the area. My obvious question, how many people had you seen have this happen to them? Her answer was quite a few, but it was years ago when these medicines were being given intravenously through peripheral veins in arms and other peripheral areas where veins are much smaller. Score 1 for the port! The process took about 20 minutes. Then she brought in a huge bag of Cyclophosamide and hung it up to go in over the next 45 minutes or so. If it ran too fast it caused a sinus headache, a really bad sinus headache.

I was beyond the point of no return. My hair would fall out in 18 days and I would start to have menopausal symptoms between the second and third treatments. Jim and I chose to sit in the movie room and watch videos. I wanted a funny one so we decided on Dr. Doolittle. Well it was funny and laughter was good and healthy. The movie and the medicine ended. The nurse cleared the port and catheter and injected more heparin into the port, to prevent clotting and I was done. I asked how soon I could expect to feel awful. No one could really say for sure but I would take the medicine just as it was prescribed. I had a lot of questions no one could answer.

Chapter 9

After Chemotherapy

It was November the 12th, a date I would never forget as long as I lived. There was nothing more frightening than having cancer and receiving chemotherapy. I felt a little funny but could not really put my finger on what it was. It was a little like my head wasn't attached to the rest of my body. I was glad I was not driving home. I was thinking that I shouldn't need to take my anti-nausea medicine until about 10:00 that evening. When I arrived home, I ate some soup and then rested, meditated, and visualized for the duration of the afternoon until the kids got home. I visualized a successful dose of chemotherapy coursing through my veins making sure there were no errant cancer cells left. I decided I would be really good to myself for a few days after chemotherapy and just rested a lot. I even prepared dinner this first day of chemotherapy and the whole family ate the same thing. As yet, I was not experiencing any nausea. This was a bit like waiting for the other shoe to drop. I knew something awful would be coming.

Things were great until about 7:00 pm. The nausea hit me like a brick. I was so nauseous. I could never have even imagined this. How could I wait until 10:00 to start the medicine? This was not stomach flu nausea. This was the worst nausea I had ever experienced. I felt awful and it came out of nowhere. One minute I was fine and the next barely able to lift my head off the pillow. I was too sick to even yell at Jim for help. Janet called me during this time. I could barely talk on the phone. I was sure I was going to vomit. I told her how sick I was and she suggested that I take the nausea medicine now. Although it was still too early to take it by the oncologist's office standards, I figured I had nothing to lose except this awful feeling so I took it and prayed. Every swallow was a challenge and I knew I had to keep the medicine down or it would not do me any good. I knew that I could not tolerate this every time I received chemotherapy. By the time I went to sleep a few hours later, I was feeling much better. Actually it took just about an hour for my stomach to feel better. It was a long hour of mind over matter. I could certainly understand why they told me to stay on top of the nausea. I was to take the medicine twice a day for three days and you can bet I would not miss a dose. I also knew to take the medicine much earlier than I had been told. I would not forget this the next time, to be sure.

From my counseling session with the nurse I knew that the first three days would be the worst, even lasting up to a week. I won't try to exercise for a few days either. I tried visualizing everyday, particularly when I knew I had chemotherapy on board, because that just made my healing 'stars' more invincible. I also prayed a lot, for myself and my family. I felt strength from all the prayers I knew were coming from all over the country. I still caught myself starting to feel anxious but I prayed instantly no matter where I was and I felt peace descend upon me like a warm cloud. I had the kids move all my scrap booking supplies upstairs to my bedroom. It was bright and sunny so I could see to work. It was also warmer than the rest of the house because of the radiant heat from the sun, and I could take frequent naps because my bed was right there beside me. I slowly started to complete some pages every day and I felt very productive.

My first chemotherapy had been on a Tuesday and it was now Saturday. I had made it through the first round. I did not miss a meal and was not nauseous after that first day. I might have quit chemotherapy if that nausea had persisted. I did have a funny, tinny, metallic taste in my mouth which lasted for about a week. I was feeling a little more empowered like I could actually get through this. I just had to keep putting one foot in front of the other and I would get through chemotherapy. It was a gorgeous autumn day and I was not going out to any of the kid's games because from now on my immune system would be deteriorating. I wanted to get away from the house and do something normal.

Chapter 10

Tragedy revisited

I decided to take a long walk the Saturday after the first treatment, and it felt great to be outside. I tried to figure out how I could simplify my life and get back to what was really important. We make life far too complicated, and I tried hard to slow the out of control spiral that had become my life. I think having cancer does that to you. Life became very precious and I refused to waste time worrying about useless things. I started to pray about how I needed to change my life. My first thought was to get a smaller house with less maintenance. The kids loved this house. We've lived here longer than anywhere else in their lives, and I've lived here longer than anywhere in my life. As part of a military family, you could not comfortably put down any roots. Maybe this was not the answer, but I knew I would eventually get the answers if I prayed for them. I knew there was something more we could do to reduce stress and simplify our lives. As I walked and contemplated, life's colors seemed more vivid. The leaves still hanging onto life were beautiful and vibrant red, yellow, and orange. Arriving home, I was invigorated.

The phone was ringing as I walked in the door from my walk. Jim was on the line and told me to sit down. He had been dong hospital rounds and he sounded very serious and upset. I was fine so he couldn't possibly have more bad news about my health. He told me that our friend and primary care doctor had dropped dead while running on a trail not far from the hospital. He had been brought by ambulance to the Emergency Department with no spontaneous heart beats or respirations. The EMT's were doing CPR. Despite desperate attempts to save his life, he was dead. Well there you have it. Life could always get worse when you thought you were as low as possible. I was grief stricken as was the whole medical community and all of the people who lived in our small town. How could I cope with this and I could only imagine the grief his family must have felt. They must be in absolute disbelief. He was our age and his children were close to our children's ages. This could have been me or Jim. Surely all the difficulties and sadness would end and there would be something positive and hopeful to take their place. I missed the wake and the funeral because I was afraid to be in such a large crowd. Jim made it to the wake and my dad attended the funeral so I felt like we had been well represented. I would get to my chance to grieve later. I would visit his grave and resolve my feelings. I did not know when I could be able to do that, but I knew that I would. At that moment, all I could do was pray for his family.

A week after chemotherapy, I felt well enough to be able to get out of the house to accomplish a few errands. Most of them were drive through places, like the bank or quick in and out stops, like the cleaners. Jim cannot take everyday off work, but I still did not want to face other people. I was able to exercise fairly well, not at my maximum effort but, I'm getting closer and I was able to do some sit-ups. I was not yet six weeks post-surgery, so I had not been given the go ahead to do anything I would like. I needed to exercise and for some reason I cried a lot when I did.

I prayed a lot and talked to my mom and to my recently departed primary care physician. I felt like I had to say some things that I never got a chance to say. I told my mom how glad I was that she did not have to go through this with me, at least not here. I thought I was finally starting to grieve my loss. I had to move so quickly into the breast cancer that I never really had a chance to deal with my mom's death. I really missed her. Initially I was angry that she left me to face this alone, but then I realized it would have killed her to see me go through breast cancer and treatment. My wonderful friends were still there through thick and thin with encouraging scripture and cards. They even still sent flowers which really brightened my day. Terri and her family sent flowers that happened to arrive the day of my first chemotherapy. I don't know if she planned it that way but I suspect she did. I did not even know how people knew what was happening. They had a special communication system. They were not calling me unless it was to tell me what time they were bringing dinner. What an absolute blessing to be in such a caring neighborhood.

My energy level was better. I seemed to only need one rest time where I actually slept. During my second rest time of the day, I meditated, visualized, or both. Most of all I was productive. I was getting a lot of scrap book pages completed and I even finished Jerred's scrapbook so I could wrap it as a Christmas present. I hoped he liked it as much as I enjoyed putting it together. It enabled me to watch him grow up and fall in love with him all over again and remember all the wonderful times. He was such a beautiful baby with big beautiful blue eyes. This was very therapeutic for me. As we faced death we could only hope that our lives had been worthwhile. Looking in the faces of my children was all that was necessary to know that we had done well.

I was coming to terms with this but I was not close to resolution. One of my most frequent prayers at that time was that I would see a reason for the suffering. Somehow in the middle of this ordeal, I realized that in order to live and be a survivor, I needed to learn to accept death, how to die. *To live, I needed to learn how to die.* This was another epiphany for me. I worked through the grief process and faced life conflicts we usually faced in old age. Working on the scrapbooks gave me the reaffirmation that my life was not in vain and I had accomplished a lot. I had a very successful military career and was in the process of raising five wonderful children. I was not done yet though. I knew I had unfinished business to attend to. I just did not know what that business was. I wanted to leave a legacy of something, and I was not sure what that might be. I considered the possibility that my legacy was already established, but I was not sure that if I were to die that I could have defined what it was. One of my prayers centered on what I could do to make a difference. Just what would be my legacy? What would I be remembered for?

For the short term, I knew that I was ready to move on to Ryan's scrapbook next. It seemed easier and logical to go from oldest to youngest. I looked forward to watching him grow and change in pictures as I had done with Jerred.

My chemotherapy slump was over for now and I was in the lowest phase of my white blood cell count, which also meant that my immune system was at its lowest point. Since this was the first time I had reached this after starting chemotherapy, I actually had to go to the lab and get blood drawn. I did not get a phone call from the doctor with the results, so I could only assume that they were fine or within normal limits as we like to say in the medical field. I wished for the next four months, I never went lower than the initial results. If a segment of the white blood cell levels were to fall too far below the normal, chemotherapy would be suspended until they rose again and I would not want that.

I wished that I was able to go to sleep and wake up without being on the verge of panic which seemed to be a recurring theme throughout my cancer ordeal. The only good thing was that prayer continued to be effective, and relieved me of much of my anxiety and gave me some peace. I had not felt like this since I was pregnant with Kate. So close to panic. I prayed hard, took deep cleansing breaths and opened my thoughts to God's comfort. I had to increase my clonazepam (tranquilizer) dosage and could not seem to wean myself off the medication for sleep, but none of my doctors seemed worried. Thanks to a friend of Jim's who became my expert alternative medicine advisor, I started on Black Cohosh for my menopausal symptoms. They would come any day but typically occurred between the second and third treatments. Specifically, I took Remifemin. My expert in alternative medicine was a retired obstetrician and gynecologist, who now taught principles of alternative medicine at the university level to medical students and physicians. It took several weeks for this herb to work so I started early so that I could reach a therapeutic level before my symptoms became more severe. I had many old wives' tales running through my brain describing the typical menopausal woman, and my mom was a screaming lunatic as I recall, but I don't know if I actually remembered very accurately. About the same time she was going through menopause, she was also diagnosed with high blood pressure and maybe all of her symptoms were a side effect of the antihypertensive medication. The medications used thirty five years ago had a very high side effect profile. She went on hormone replacement therapy (HRT) for her menopausal symptoms, and continued on it until the day she died. HRT would not be an option for me because the hormones could cause an estrogen sensitive cancer like mine to reactivate.

I had cut out all the antioxidants in my vitamin therapy as well as the calcium supplement. The reason for this was that I did not want to be in such good shape that the chemotherapy was unable to kill the cancer cells. Basically, I did not want to be a suitable host to cancer cells, so I had to take good care of me but not the cancer cells. The calcium was just hard to digest while undergoing chemotherapy. I felt very vulnerable to disease. As soon as chemotherapy was over, my alternative care doctor would help me select the appropriate nutritional supplements for maximum health. I was only two weeks into this regimen with ten weeks to go. I was feeling far too wise before my time. Becoming an expert on breast cancer had never been my intention. Facing death had certainly made me very philosophical. I took one baby step at a time and the time was going so slowly. I prayed that each chemotherapy session would be no worse that the last and I could keep my life as normal as possible, which was my best medicine.

Next week was Thanksgiving. Traditionally before we bless our food we ask what everyone at the table was thankful for. I asked that we not do this on Thanksgiving Day this year because I knew I would start crying uncontrollably. I had so much to be thankful for. I cannot begin to recite my blessings nor number them. My husband Jim and my family were so supportive that I could not imagine going through any of this without them. God had not left my side through any part of this. I felt sorry for my dad as this was just so difficult for him with so many events happening in rapid succession, but he too, continued his daily visits to my house. Up until October, he was not even able to drive. It took so long for him to recover after surgery. Driving was something he cherished as a symbol of his independence. Jerred would be coming home the following week. I could not wait to see him. He had become my good buddy the previous summer when we had so much time to spend together before he left for college. I thought when he saw me, he would be reassured that I was doing just fine and he would realize he had nothing to worry about. College was what he should worry about right now, not his mother's health.

Chapter 11

Hair Free, Care Free

Just before Thanksgiving Geri came to visit for a day during the weekend as she had done every weekend since my surgery. She always brought a meaningful card and usually a gift of a book or CD. This time she had something else. It was not any package I had seen before. My curiosity was certainly piqued and she was very excited. We had talked about a store in Loveland that had hats and wigs for people on chemotherapy, but she actually went to the store and talked to the owner. She handed me a gift bag with a cute hat with a decorative band and bangs for me. Not noises, but bangs like those in your hair. This was such a thoughtful gift and I had not begun to deal with the fact that my hair was going to fall out soon. I only knew that day was coming faster than I wanted. We tried on the hat and bangs and it looked real. Furthermore, the hat was very flattering and cute. With bangs on your forehead and a hat no one could tell whether you have hair or not. This was going to happen and I better think about it. What was it with women and hair? The fact that it would all fall out was somehow mortifying. I decided to become proactive and ordered some other simple little hats. I looked at wigs but was not too thrilled with what I saw in catalogs but, I decided I would at least look at the wig store in Loveland to try on a few, some other day. I would at least give a wig a chance.

That night after my shower I noticed the floor of the shower was covered with hair. I do not remember noticing all that hair before. Over the next week, I started to get a funny prickly, itchy feeling on my scalp. The oncology nurse had warned me that I would be able to tell when my hair would fall out. That prickly feeling was the hair as it became detached at the follicle. Since hair cells rapidly duplicated, it was one of the first affected by the chemotherapy. It sometimes came out in clumps when I rubbed my hands through my hair. I looked at my hands and shuddered at the amount of hair. It was like looking at a lot of blood all over my hands.

This was Thanksgiving week, and we traditionally had my sister take our Christmas Photo for our Christmas card. I asked Jim if we would be sending a photo or even cards. I thought a New Years card without a picture might be a bit more optimistic since I would be finishing with the chemotherapy in January. I lost the argument. I chose not to deal with the card at all. He wrote it as always.

Actually he did everything with the card including signing all of mine and addressing the envelopes and mailing them. Although I looked forward to the holidays, this year I could not bear to write any notes on any cards. The card was painful for me to read.

Every night after my shower I checked how much hair had fallen out. It's everywhere. It covered the vanity when I dried it with the dryer and when I just combed it. It was a very humiliating experience. All of it should fall out at once... It was torture to watch it come out by bits and pieces. To look at me though, you really can't tell that it's falling out. We have a lot of hair and can lose a lot before others notice. I was reminded of the years that I used to pull my hair out as a nervous habit. Hopefully, that would be part of history when this was over and I had hair again. That too, seemed a very long way off. On Thanksgiving morning after seeing how much hair was on my pillow, I woke up and told Jim that I wanted to cut my hair off right away. Of course he refused to do it and I started to cry. He wanted me to wait until Jerred arrived this morning so we could pose for pictures. I felt ugly and I did not want to be in a picture. Then he asked that I just get through the day and Thanksgiving dinner before he would shave the hair off for me. The anticipation drove me crazy all day. I was obsessed with shaving my head as soon as possible. Janet was here to cook the whole meal and we were expecting guests, as well as dad. I had a very hard time dealing with the first Thanksgiving without my mom so I disappeared by myself to have another good cry. I was afraid to live with this disease and afraid I might die from it. I was afraid to lose my hair and afraid of all the effects of the chemotherapy and other medication that I knew would come. I did almost nothing to help with the dinner. I found myself immobilized with the events of my life. It was hard to keep a stiff upper lip with everyone.

Dinner was great but I really just wanted the day to be over. Janet took my dad home and then returned. Jim, Janet, and Jerred together got ready to shave all my hair off. There were a lot of tears and some pretty funny moments as I thought about having my husband, son, and sister shave all my hair off. I even thought to take a picture as I just sat there as the hair fell to the floor. Was that really my hair? It was hard to tell through the tears. The hair looked so dark. Was my hair really that dark? Janet did not understand how it looked so dark on the floor and light on my head. The first thing I noticed after becoming hair free was how cold my head was. I was freezing. I took a shower and washed my hair which was odd since I had no hair, but I went through the motions just the same. I was still freezing after the shower. Luckily I had ordered a night hat, never really thinking I might need one. Kate called it my angel hat. There was an angel embroidered on the front of the hat. It was made of soft cotton and I put it on and was instantly warm. Score a big win for hats. I was never able to look at myself in the mirror that night. I suddenly had a new appreciation for bald men. They must be cold a lot or develop a very tough scalp. A few more tears and I was able to sleep.

When I awakened, I forgot that my hair was gone, briefly, since my head was warm. I went into the bathroom and slowly took my hat off in front of the mirror. There, staring back at me was a hairless head and I quickly put on the hat and bangs that Geri gave me. Janet, Geri, and I planned a trip to the wig store in Loveland. I was curious now that I had heard so much about the store and the owner Frieda. We had planned all along, to go on the Friday after Thanksgiving. I did not think this was what most shoppers planned to do on the biggest shopping day of the year and the traditional start to the Christmas shopping season. I was still supposed to have my hair so we could match colors, but luckily I had taken some Polaroid photos before I shaved the hair off so we would have a good idea for color. After all it was not the same color it should have been anyway. Maybe I should just get a black wig and really shock everyone. We arrived at the wig store which also happened to be a Christian bookstore right at 10:00 am when they opened. It was an unusual mix of items in the same store. It was a good thing we arrived early as it got busy very quickly. We waited for Frieda to arrive. We all tried on a couple of wigs. Then we started to look through the hats and decorative bands. I experienced a few near tear moments. Janet and Geri made it so much fun trying on so many wigs.

When Frieda arrived, she sat me down and took off my hat. Wow, there I was in this store with huge mirrors and bright lights sitting in a styling chair with people staring at me and I had no hair. This was the first time I had examined my head without hair. My reflection stared back at me from every mirror. I was bald. What a shock! I was so close to tears but everyone tried to be as jovial as possible to keep my spirits up. I was sure that I tried on every wig in the store. They were coming at me from all sides. There were long ones, short ones, curly ones, and all different colored ones. I had to admit it was a bit like a fantasy, being able to change what I looked like so quickly. Janet, Frieda, and Geri all picked out wigs. We finally settled on one although there were three that I could have walked out of the store with and been very happy. I ordered one that we all thought was the perfect color. Then the three ladies started with the hats and had me in every hat style with a different decorative band. This was actually almost fun. Shaving off my hair was certainly better than waiting for it to fall out on its own, but I still had cancer and was still devastated, but I was being proactive.

Now I thought I had survived the worst of the hair falling out, I thought that I had really jumped a huge hurdle. Then as I was getting ready to take a shower, I started to notice that my pubic hair was thinning. I was certain no one told me that *all* my hair would fall out. It ultimately all fell out. I now looked like a prepubescent twelve year old. This was the ultimate in humiliation. I could deal with not having to shave my legs and arms. That was a nice side effect. I thought I was told that pubic hair might fall out, not that it would fall out. I tried to listen during my patient teaching appointment. At least I still had eyebrows and eye lashes, which surprised me a lot.

My exercise time got longer and more normal and I felt stronger. I continued to meditate and pray several times a day. I was still afraid I was going to die but everyone involved in my care was very optimistic. Prayer got me through each and every minute. I was always on the verge of tears. I usually started a conversation with, "Don't be too nice to me or I will cry." That caught people before they asked me anything. Friends learned quickly not to start a conversation asking me how I was. I reminded my doctors each time I visited. I was living in self imposed isolation, partly because I did not want to get sick and partly because I just could not deal with this cancer face to face and I still felt like a freak. I found the time alone to be one of enlightenment. I tried to purge all bad thoughts. I loved getting the scrap booking done and I had quality time with God all day. I knew that to look at me most people would not think I was sick but I felt like it was tattooed on my forehead. "I have breast cancer." Now that I felt better and stronger, it was time for the second barrage with chemotherapy which was the week after Thanksgiving. That was great timing. I felt very good physically over the holiday and I was ready to be half way through the chemotherapy.

Jim took me in again for the second treatment. I got my blood drawn and they checked my weight. I've lost a little less than five pounds but not enough to recalculate the medication dosage. I saw the doctor as I always must because he made sure that I was healthy enough for chemotherapy. He was also quite proud of me for having shaved my hair off and I was really stylish with a hat today. My granulocytes (a fraction of my white blood cells) were at 1.6. 1.5 was the cut off low for getting chemotherapy. A few weeks ago I had my nadir blood drawn. That was the day during the cycle of chemotherapy that the white blood cell count was at its lowest. It occurred about 10 days after chemotherapy. My blood levels had not changed at all since then, which surprised me because I believed I would rebound very quickly because I was in such good shape. I visualized my 'stars' wiping out all the cancer cells and visualized my bone marrow pumping out big strong white cells. It seemed like I was unable to help my body fight the side effects and I felt like it was a setback. I felt like a failure. I did not like to feel this helpless.

Chemotherapy tended to be cumulative in its effect so I had to see what this next dose would do. I was better prepared for the events to come this time. Jim and I still chose to watch a funny movie while I received treatment. It was much like a date except the room was about 50 degrees and we sat in two separate chairs. Still, it was time together that I was not sure I would have forever. This time they had to access my port. That was a little uncomfortable when they stuck the needle in. The needle was at a 90 degree angle and very odd looking. The port was the one thing that I found to be really uncomfortable. It stuck out just below my right collar bone and rubbed on everything; seat belt, clothing, and everything else. The chemotherapy all went in and my urine turned red almost instantaneously. This time as the medication infused I tried to visualize the chemotherapy going through my body wiping away all the cancer cells wherever they might be if there were any left. The chairs in the Cancer Center were some of the most comfortable around and once I got enough blankets on, I was downright cozy. There were some beautiful quilts in the center that people had made and donated. We were done about noon and went home to start the whole cycle all over again. The entire process took about half the day. It seemed like it should go faster but it could not.

I was back to resting for the two days after chemotherapy thinking it would give the chemotherapy a better chance to work, plus the treatment tired me out. The cycle was becoming quite clear. First, I felt good. Then I received chemotherapy and felt washed out and fatigued for a week. The second week I began to feel better but had the tinny taste in my mouth. By week three, I felt pretty good and much stronger just in time for the cycle to start again. This time I knew to take the anti-nausea medicine earlier, before I felt sick. I learned very quickly that the nausea of chemotherapy was miserable. My spiritual relationship kept me going. God was still right beside me. I prayed for peace and He was right there with me helping me feel it. The next few weeks would bring the first signs of menopause. It was funny how everyone in oncology knew the exact day the various side effects occurred. I hoped the Black Cohosh would have the desired effect and would decrease the menopausal symptoms, particularly the hot flashes. I braced for the worst and hoped for the best. I was certain I was going to have every single bad symptom that any research had uncovered. That was very pessimistic, but I still seemed to be in a cycle where if anything could go wrong; it would.

Chapter 12

Six Weeks Post-Op

Three days after the second chemotherapy treatment was my 6 week post-operative appointment with the plastic surgeon. Six weeks was the magical time after major surgery when most problems disappeared and you could return to normal activities. The plastic surgeon was still ecstatic with the way my breasts turned out and even took pictures this visit. I was happy to start her book of photographs for patients to see examples of her work. The new breasts were a bit uncomfortable but I hated to make her feel bad. I sometimes wished I did not have the new breasts. I received the go ahead to exercise as tolerated and to sleep on my stomach. The most exciting news was that I did not have to stuff a sanitary napkin in the side of my bra anymore and tape it all up. I had taken a few liberties with exercise anyway. It was a relief to have no restrictions. I still felt like I had football shoulder pads on. I did not know if it was caused by the numb areas on my chest and back or by my seemingly huge new breasts. Unfortunately, doing some very mild push-ups, I popped a little hernia at the top of my right breast. It was my fault and I knew I had done too much, too soon.

The second visit with the psychiatrist was easier, since she wanted to make sure that I was not having problems with the upcoming holidays. I really did not need a psychiatrist. I was in total control of my emotions, much better than the last time I saw her. I was in my wig and she asked if I had lost my hair. That was a good sign if she could not tell the difference. Of course, she did not know me very well and had seen me only once before. I told her that I had shaved my head rather than wait for the hair to fall out.

She seemed happy to know that I had decorated for Christmas and gotten my shopping done, most of which I did before surgery. I assured her that I was looking forward to the holidays despite the cancer. She seemed happy and fairly secure that I was not depressed enough to kill myself, since that would not have reflected well on her. That of course, was the reason I needed to see her in the first place. I left and did not have to return unless something changed. Finally I could get rid of one doctor. Seeing them all was taking up so much valuable time. I was sure the insurance company had good reasons for insisting I see a psychiatrist, but I was not a psychiatrist person. Thank goodness those two visits were over.

The tears still continued to come frequently, and I was sure that I was beginning to grieve for my mother now that I had time to think about her. I also grieved for the loss of my breasts and for the potential loss of my own life. I felt that this was all pretty healthy. I was sure I was also grieving for the loss of my child bearing years. This was quite a lot to deal with all at the same time. I had quite a few hot flashes now, and I was awakened several times a night in a pool of sweat. Other than that I did not think I had any other symptoms. I was grateful that was all that I felt. I had not become depressed or lost my libido and I was not at all irritable. At least that was my perspective. If it never got worse than this I would be fine.

Just before the holidays I began listening to K-LOVE, a Christian radio station. There were no commercials and it was very positive. I found it to be very uplifting and it kept me centered on what was important, particularly now during the holidays. Listening to Christian Christmas music helped me really stay focused on the reason we celebrated Christmas. More than any other time in my life, this Advent I was really spending time waiting and praying. I worked on the scrapbooks and got daily sunshine. I could look out and rejoice at the beauty that God gave us. I felt like I was resolving all of my grief. Christmas was coming and I did not know how I would be as the holiday got closer. I hated to look at this as my last Christmas because I thought I had many more to come. I remembered my message when I was lying on the couch, about not dying. I was pretty confident.

My friend Suzi was getting ready to leave for the holidays and fly to Hawaii with her family, but before she left, she sent me a gift with Erik. It was a book by Stormie Omartian, The Power of a Praying Woman. I had read many of her books but this one gave a woman permission to pray for herself. This was not all that earth shattering but it was a pivotal point for me in my life. I had always prayed for everyone else and now I felt I could and should pray for myself and not feel guilty. I could pray to be a better parent and to reject satan and to understand the path that God was directing me toward. This seemed to open up a new world for me. I tried to spend time reading the book every day but not too much because I loved the book so much that I did not want to finish it. The Christmas holidays were coming and so was chemotherapy. Jerred was also coming home for the holidays. I felt so good before chemotherapy, at least relatively speaking, that it was always hard to prepare myself for the next round of treatment knowing I would not feel very good for several days after it was completed. In some strange way it was like working out. It might be uncomfortable at the time but the benefits came later.

Jerred arrived home earlier than usual for his Christmas break; just a coincidence of how the holidays fell that year. He was able to take me to my next chemotherapy appointment. I felt good about the upcoming controlled poisoning. It was my third treatment of four and I would be three quarters of the way done. The nausea was controlled by medication and although I was not breezing through this period in my life, it could have been much worse. Jerred accompanied me to chemotherapy two days before Christmas. I was not too worried because I had weathered the two previous treatments fairly well. The office was decorated for the holidays and the decorations were very dignified, so politically correct, considering it was an oncology clinic. They had a tree but no reference to Jesus' birth anywhere.

We arrived and I signed in and paid my co-pay just like always and they called me to draw my blood. This was just like it had been at the previous appointments. My own physician was on vacation but I was scheduled to see another physician in the same group. I knew that, so it did not come as a surprise to me. What was a surprise when I got into the exam room was my white blood cell count and granulocyte count. They even repeated the test and the levels were simply too low to give me chemotherapy. The doctor delivered the bad news. Nobody mentioned that this might be a possibility. I was quite aware that my immune system was seriously compromised. I was absolutely devastated and I held the substitute physician personally responsible. I was so upset but tried not to cry in front of this stranger. I asked if there was any way I could receive chemotherapy. The answer was no. The doctor asked if I had been on any medication to stimulate white blood cells. No, I was not and this doctor was not going to change anything. I hated this man. I left for home feeling awful. No one told me that this could happen although I should have known. The nurse in me was on vacation and I was not really thinking clearly or intelligently. I was so depressed and of course everyone called to see how the third treatment had gone. They were as disappointed as I was, especially Janet and Geri. Christmas was in two days and I did not want to ruin the day for everyone. I shed a lot more tears and wondered how and why this happened to me. Wasn't it enough that I had cancer in the first place? Why in the world would the treatment schedule have to be altered now? My schedule was now off and I would not be done by January 12th as I had previously planned.

My need to control was rearing its ugly head. What was wrong with me? What was wrong with my visualization technique? I tried to do it everyday. I just knew I was doing something wrong. God had something else to say to me. He was in control. I was not in control. For whatever reason I needed to wait for the next chemotherapy until after Christmas. It was disappointing but I needed to get over it so my family could enjoy Christmas. I did not want to beat myself with guilt. I prayed and prayed and finally found some peace even if it was a bit tenuous.

The next day was Christmas Eve. We made all the final preparations for the holiday. My neighbor Carol, who was a gourmet cook, was bringing us a turkey. It was more than I could ever ask. I was so grateful. She brought it on Christmas Eve instead of Christmas Day because I did not want to interfere with her family's holiday. My neighbor Linda brought the rest of the dinner. My family left for the Christmas Eve service at church. I had not missed a service in as long as I could remember. I had no immune system so there was no way I could be in a small church packed with hundreds of people. Suddenly I started to feel really sorry for myself. No mother, (since I had just lost her), and I was all alone on the night before Christmas. I had breast cancer and I was in the middle of my chemotherapy treatments. Poor, poor me. As I sat watching the twinkling lights on the Christmas tree, the phone rang. I was tempted not to answer because I was not in a talkative mood at all. However, I did answer and it was Geri. She knew that I had been crying. I was so glad she called and talked to me and kept me company through the rest of the time my family was gone. Her timing was perfect. That really did not surprise me too much. She had a sixth sense. I got out of self pity mode. I managed to put on a happy face and enjoy the delicious feast with my family.

Despite the circumstances we were able to have a fairly normal Christmas Eve and Christmas Day. There were a few rough moments when I looked around at the family and wondered how many more days like this I could expect. This was all part of learning to die so that I could live. The Christmas tree seemed more beautiful than ever and I just stared at the twinkling lights that reminded me of the stars in the sky. I was able to transcend the clamor of Christmas morning and watch briefly from a distance: my wonderful children, the joy and laughter on their faces and all the colorful wrappings and presents. Again it was like watching a movie. It was a beautiful sight and I really enjoyed just watching but I wanted to be part of it too, so I came back to reality and we all had a great time opening presents and playing with them. This year it seemed a lot easier to concentrate and share the joy of the true meaning of Christmas; the birth of our Lord and Savior, Jesus Christ. Sure, the gifts were there but so was the love and support of my family which second to Jesus' birth is the greatest gift of all. In the infamous words of Lou Gehrig, I felt like *the luckiest person in the world*. What an absolute blessing.

The Cancer Center scheduled me to return two days after Christmas for another blood test and possibly chemotherapy. Jim was able to go to this appointment with me. I was afraid to get my hopes up because I had no idea whether my immune system was strong enough for this next insult. This was session three of four again, so I was really excited to be getting so close to the end. I got my blood drawn and the nurse immediately sent us back to the treatment area. I thought this was a good sign. They must think that I would be able to receive the treatment or they would not have sent me back to the treatment room. I did not get too comfortable under the blankets or put another movie in until I was sure we would be staying. This process was a series of ups and downs, joys and disappointments. It was so painful and yet I was learning so much about myself. We waited anxiously and finally saw the nurse come in with a big grin. I squeaked by again and would get the total dose of medication. My white blood cell counts were barely within the range of being able to receive chemotherapy. Sometimes if the counts were low, they would administer a smaller dose of the chemotherapy. That would feel like defeat to me. I never in my life thought there would be a day that I would be so excited to get chemotherapy, but I was today. This was a small victory, but a victory nonetheless. Something was finally going right. This time we were in and out in a bit over an hour. I was so happy to have more of the day to spend at home with my family.

I was in for a rude awakening because this time I had a throbbing sinus headache. I searched my memory banks for a reason for this, since I had not ever had a headache before. Rapid infusion of cyclophosamide could cause a severe sinus headache. Sure enough the headache persisted for about 24 hours, but I got through it the best I could with a lot of acetaminophen. I really understood how to take the medication for the nausea so this time I had no nausea.

I had asked this nurse, who was new to me when we were getting treatment, about the tamoxifen after chemotherapy. Tamoxifen blocks the estrogen my body produced which my tumor had thrived on. I was a bit obsessed with this. She said to tough it out for a month and that would be the worst of it. If I felt like my husband was driving me crazy and I wanted to kill him that was normal and to call the nurse triage line and tell them about it. Oh, I felt really good now. She also said to take heart because I would be going through, in a month, what it took most women several years to go through. Namely menopause. I guessed there was something to be said for that. Again I tried to rest for a few days after chemotherapy, hoping that if I did not tax my body with superfluous things, I would help the chemotherapy be more effective.

I was doing really well on my scrap booking project and it was such fun putting our lives together in photos and mementos. I looked so forward to working on them everyday. I prayed a lot every day for myself and my family and my situation and for peace. I started to read the Bible everyday as well. I just opened it and started reading. It was such a therapeutic time for me. I don't know when or how it happened, but I knew why. I had really let God take control and lead me where He wanted me. I started to resolve many issues in my mind. All the uncertainty and the agonizing finally became easier to deal with. This could only be an answer to my prayers. God's hand was all over these feelings. If I were to die from this cancer, I realized that my life had been very worthwhile.

The years came rushing back to me. I had and still have a very successful career. This had always been the most difficult hurdle for me because I didn't continue working full time after my children were born, and I always wondered what it would be like now if I had continued to work. I had made a difference, though. I had touched the lives of thousands of people. Through nursing school and my years as a nurse both full and part time there were people who would not have been around without me. That was an accomplishment not everyone could claim. I had been the last person some of my patients ever saw. Those were difficult moments but the families were always somehow happier knowing that their loved ones were not alone. I had made a pact with myself early in my career that God would help me and I would never let anyone die alone. That was a blessing too. I was glad I was able to do that much. Although I felt like I was a movie character, it was important for me to have these visions come back to me as an answer to my prayer that I had made a difference and my life had been very meaningful. I left a legacy. I was coming face to face with my mortality. I was finally able to complete grieving for my mother and for my primary care physician. The tears streamed down my face daily, as I dealt with these realizations, I felt like I was being purged. Many tears were those of unequaled joy. My mother was in a better place and was free from all her illnesses and she was perfect in heaven. My primary care physician would never know the potential pain of growing old. He would never know the pain of cancer or a debilitating illness. Through my own experiences both working and losing a child at her birth, I had developed a philosophy of death that allowed me to see God in the senseless deaths of children. They never experienced any hardships and they never experienced pain. They never knew the ugly side of life and their lives were perfect. God had chosen them to come back to Him sooner than we would like. A neighbor of mine and good friend of my family wrote me not long after Mary, our daughter, died, and described a beautiful scene to me that I would cherish always. That was Jesus, against a beautiful sunset carrying my baby girl away with Him. It was a vision of tremendous peace.

I would be lucky to die quickly and there were benefits in that for all of us. I preferred not to go now, however. I realized that I could die right now and I would be at peace. I knew there was a heaven and knew God was there. This was my defining moment and I was extremely aware because I learned how to die and a part of me had died. I mourned the loss of my very naive life, but was enlightened by how I wanted to live the rest of my life however long that might be. Once this revelation became clear to me, I was able to move ahead and look forward to my life. I was experiencing how to live again. I could not imagine a life without God. Did I see God's presence in all that I was going through? Absolutely! The issues I was dealing with and praying about were stages that I had to progress through successfully. This was a personal journey that God was taking me on, and one that would result in my becoming a better Christian and a better person. No one could accompany me on this journey. I could not even share these most intimate revelations with my family. This was between my God and me. I did not believe I had ever had such clarity of thought and of God.

Not long after the holidays I received a letter from a college classmate and friend. Her name was Deb. She had been diagnosed with breast cancer just before Christmas and was not sure where she was headed because she had not met with all the physicians. I was shocked but a little relieved that I would have someone to share this with. I thought if I kept in touch with other cancer survivors, I could create my own support group. Doctors and nurses reminded me often that I should be part of a support group, but I could not bring myself to participate in such a group. I knew Deb wasn't relieved by her diagnosis but I resolved to keep writing to her during what ended up being 6 months of chemotherapy and radiation. I really wanted to uplift her as much as my friends were able to do the same for me. She and her family were a part of my daily prayers.

I had a routine follow up appointment with my general surgeon. I had not seen her since she put my port in because I was followed so closely by the plastic surgeon and the oncologist. I saw her every three months for two visits and then every six months. She seemed very happy with my progress and taught me how to do self breast exams with all the new muscle and implants. It most definitely felt different than before the surgery. I still could not let up on this aspect of my health. Monthly self breast exams were still critical. Diligence and knowing what you were feeling was so important. Frequent follow up appointments with the doctors were invaluable. They helped me to know what was normal. The doctor assured me that the greatest incidence of recurrence of a breast tumor would be superficial and easy to palpate and would most likely occur within the first two years. I did not need a yearly mammogram any more. I tried to set up a time to get my port out but I realized I was rushing things since my immune system took such a long time to bounce back after chemotherapy. I needed to be patient. Now I'm hoping to have my last chemotherapy on the 16th of January. I had thought the oncologist said I could get the port out right away but my right away was the 17th of January. I did not think that was what he had in mind. No surgeon wanted to electively take an immunosuppressed patient into the operating room. The port couldn't come out soon enough for me. When I looked at it I felt like I was a sick person and I did not want to be a sick person. The general surgeon did not deliver a clean bill of health, but things did look better and she felt no new lumps or bumps. I had to be happy with very small steps. I would see her again in April for a regular appointment, but knew I'd have my port out a few months before that, and she would remove it.

My days seemed very full between exercising, meditating, visualizing, reading my Bible, resting, and continuing with my scrapbooks for the kids. After the completion of many pages, my supplies were running very low and I needed to get reinforcements. I resolved not to count the pages I finished because I did not want that pressure, and not knowing the exact number of pages I had completed was just fine. Ordinarily I would count everyday to monitor my progress. I was trying to get rid of stress in my life for good. Counting the number of pages I completed would be counterproductive to what I tried to teach myself and prayed about and that was reducing my anxiety. Through prayer I thought I was successfully doing just that.

The next three weeks seemed to drag by, but, I knew it would take everything in me to boost my immune system so that I could get the next and final treatment completed. It was so close but not here yet. I stayed as busy as I could and did not stress about anything. Right after my next treatment was scheduled was a long weekend. Jim would be gone with Justin and Kate at a soccer tournament in Orlando, Florida. It would be Kate's first visit to Disneyworld. They were all very excited, but I needed to find someone to take me to chemotherapy. Janet and Geri would both be here for the long weekend and to celebrate with me the end of my controlled poisoning. I had hoped to feel good and be able to really enjoy the visit. Neither one would be here for the actual treatment, so I called on my friend Mary Lou to take me to the treatment. At this point, I felt strong and optimistic, and having someone with me was not as necessary as it had been earlier in my treatments. Dependence on others was difficult, but my friend Mary Lou was delighted to help by taking me to the cancer center.

Chapter 13

The Final Chemotherapy

Just before the long weekend celebrating Martin Luther King's birthday, Jim, Justin, and Kate took an early flight on their way to Florida, and I looked so forward to the final appointment. I knew better than to think anything was ever final. I always felt a little funny before and after chemotherapy and didn't trust myself driving. We arrived and I was called right back to have my blood drawn. I was so excited that I could hardly contain myself. I told everyone about this being the last chemotherapy for me. I got on the scale for a weight check. I had lost about twenty pounds. This was a result of my very healthy diet and not related to skipping meals or vomiting due to the chemotherapy. I felt great, but I hadn't been this skinny since I was in High School although I had never actually had a weight problem, except in college with the freshman 15. Those were the fifteen pounds freshmen could plan to put on during their first year. I figured when I went on tamoxifen I would start to gain weight and look really matronly. That was supposed to happen in menopause anyway. At least that was what everyone told me about the drug, tamoxifen. Although I was not particularly vain I did like my new weight and dreaded getting heavier and looking like an older woman. I do not want facial hair, age spots and all the afflictions that go with menopause. I had to deal with first things first though, and as I sat in the doctor's office and got checked in, I asked to see my lab results.

Usually the nursing staff makes you wait for the doctor to tell you that information, but they knew I would look at my chart anyway. My heart sank. This was one of those difficult problems with knowing too much. I did not wait for someone to give me the results, I sought them out. Once again my white cell count and granulocyte count was too low to get the medication. I saw my own oncologist this time too, so I couldn't blame the substitute doctor, not that it had been rational to do that anyway. Maybe when the oncologist came in he would have a different take on this or have a solution. This was only wishful thinking and in my heart I knew that. I hoped and prayed that the final dose of chemotherapy could be given. The doctor however, wanted me to wait until Tuesday. I convinced him Monday was better for me even though it was a holiday. Janet and Geri would both be here then and not on Tuesday. The office would be open even though the oncologist would not be working.

I could not express the disappointment and betrayal that I felt about having to deal with yet another setback. My body was not handling this chemotherapy as well as I had been sure that it would. I did everything right and things still did not turn out like I planned. I always felt as if I were invincible. My immune system was just taking too much of a beating. Then I asked if I could still get my port out on February 13th as I had planned. Actually, I originally planned to get the port removed by the 17th of January. This wasn't going to work either because he wanted to see me on February 17th before I got the port removed. I asked if I could schedule it for the 20th. He said he thought that day would be a safer bet.

I would start the dreaded tamoxifen on the 17th after I saw the oncologist again. In the midst of all the cancer, you just want to be able to look ahead at milestones that you can mark off. Although, in the grand scheme, the little events were minor, they became larger than life and a bit blown out of proportion. I decided to try, yet again, to get the real scoop on tamoxifen so I asked the oncologist to tell me about this drug. This was also a diversionary tactic to avoid thinking about my disappointment. As long as I stayed in the office, there was still a chance that I would somehow get the chemotherapy. The tamoxifen had so many side effects I still probably don't know them all. This drug affected those women who were premenopausal the most. That was me. Uterine cancer was probably the most frightening of the side effects. The chance of developing a malignancy was fairly small but I needed to be followed closely by either an ultrasound or endometrial biopsy when I got my yearly Pap smear. The other side effects were vaginal dryness, hot flashes and mild weight gain. It catapulted those women close to menopause into menopause. I worried about becoming a psychotic mess as a result of the medicine and menopause. There were some medications that might help. One of them had already been prescribed for me. That was vanlafaxine HCl. I was willing to stay on that for as long as necessary. I was also on the herbal supplement black cohosh. Both of these were to help with the hot flashes, which seemingly were the worst side effect since you had them all day and night thereby interrupting sleep and causing irritability. There were other drugs like the belladonnas and Neurontin that might help too. These two drugs have more side effects than I chose to deal with until I knew exactly how I would react to the tamoxifen. The total lack of control I had over my life made me crazy.

This would not be the weekend that I had looked forward to and planned with great anticipation. We were all here with nothing to celebrate. Janet decided to arrive on Saturday since she would like to be around for the chemotherapy instead of planning to leave on the day of my next appointment. It was hard for me to give up control but God was working very carefully trying to make me realize that I was not in control. God was definitely in control and He had a way of letting me know it.

Geri came as planned since she had made these plans at the expense of other much more exciting things she could have been doing. She brought down Mahi Mahi and Salmon. One of my healthy diet changes was to add more fish to our diets. Geri was trying very hard to teach me to cook fish that tasted good and not like fish. She seemed to be succeeding and even convinced the kids to like it. They were starting to like fish, especially the fish she cooked for them. I got over the disappointment of not receiving the final chemotherapy and we planned a nice girl's weekend even though Ryan and Erik were here. It was like a three night sleepover. Her meals were terrific. I did not help much with the meals but watched carefully. We turned the lights down and lit candles so we had some ambiance with dinner. The boys even liked the atmosphere. We giggled and talked like teenagers. She paraffin waxed my hands and my feet, which felt like warm mud oozing through my fingers and toes. That felt very strange and my skin felt great. Geri thought my hands were as soft as a baby's behind. One of the really nice side effects of the chemotherapy was the fact that like cancer cells, skin cells were also rapidly producing, so my skin cells were turning over fairly quickly and therefore my face looked great and my skin was very soft. I thought she might be a little bit jealous. I did not recommend the method but the effect was very nice. We saw Janet briefly on Sunday. She added a lot of levity and love and would pick us both up in the morning to go to the appointment.

I tried to temper both Geri and Janet's excitement with the possibility that I still might not be able to receive the chemotherapy. They wanted to hear nothing of that. Janet spent that night with my dad and Geri and I continued with the girl's weekend. I thought she needed this break because she fell asleep earlier than I did every night. Geri had always been the night owl. I was the one who needed all the sleep. This had been the case for as long as I remembered being friends, which was about 34 years and counting. My dogs Courage and Sable slept with her each night. She got a big kick out of that until they woke her up really early. We all rested extremely well, even the boys. I think we all needed the time to relax.

Janet arrived to pick us up Monday. The appointment was later than normal because they had to squeeze me in. I was afraid it would be really crowded but it was still quite calm although busier than the previous times I had come earlier in the morning. I looked around at all the people waiting for their treatments and wondered what their stories might be. What stage of cancer were they in? Do they feel like I do? Had they come to terms with their diseases and their lives? Had they been through the same things as I had? We arrived early for the appointment so we waited quietly in the waiting room awhile for the lab technicians to call me back to get my blood work done.

When Janet goes anywhere she brings everything she could possibly need to work so she looked as though she was moving in for days. While we were in the waiting room she started to read the morning paper. She started to tell us stories of the Middle East and her visits there. The war in Iraq was looming and the paper was full of stories about the build up of forces, but for some reason she was able to tell the funniest stories about her antics when she visited frequently a few years ago. Even another woman who was waiting was laughing and enjoyed the tales. They finally called me back to get my blood drawn. Again they put us right into my favorite room with the movies. This was the moment of truth. Janet took a fair amount of time trying to move all her stuff into the room and of course we had to rearrange the room to fit all of us in there, but no one cared. It was a little crowded but we were just laughing despite the air of uncertainty that hung over us. Although it was unspoken, I was very apprehensive while waiting to see the nurse walk in. She walked in shortly with a smile on her face, too. My lab work was fine and we proceeded with the final dose of chemotherapy! I explained to the nurse about the sinus headache the last time and she agreed that the medication probably infused too fast so she would slow it down this time. Now we can really move in and pick out our funny movie. Janet unloaded all her junk and her computer. She had some work to do but also had catalogs from the last month of mail so we had lots to look at. The mood was very upbeat and my port was still patent which I was always concerned about. I was always afraid it might form a clot and not be useable.

The nurse started the chemotherapy and we just settled in. Janet took out her cuticle cream and made us all put it on our cuticles. Apparently she needed to do her nails and tried to get both of us to join her. She started to file her nails and got out her nail polish. It was a pretty winter day outside and the view from the big windows was quite lovely.

In about an hour she decided that we needed to eat since its lunch time so she went down to the cafeteria, a place we knew all too well having spent a lot of time there last summer when our dad was hospitalized. My medicine was going in so slowly that I turned it up faster. Janet came back with healthy salads for lunch and some kind of vitamin drink that we couldn't open. We tried everything and just could not open the plastic bottles. Just then the nurse came in. We enlisted her help opening the bottles. By this time we were giggling about these silly bottles and our inability to get them open. After a try with little forceps and scissors the nurse finally opened them using her bandage scissors, which she cleaned with alcohol before she used them to pry off the lids on the bottles of our drinks. I again had to turn up the IV with the medicine in it because we were coming up on about two hours and the bag was not even half empty yet. I certainly did not have a sinus headache this time. The movie was long over and we were about to help Janet with her work. She had spent more time talking than working but this was a glorious day in my book.

I finally received all the medication and the nurse arrived with a coffee mug that said *Yippee*. This was my gift for having received my final chemotherapy. I loved it and it was very appropriate. I briefly thought about the people that got their yippee cups but did not survive. They could still say yippee that chemotherapy was over. Sometimes you had to celebrate the really small accomplishments. Not everyone would be a survivor. We got home about 2:00 that afternoon. Geri had to go back that night after dinner and Janet was planning to stay with me in case I had any problems. She did not want me to be alone after chemotherapy. I assured her I was probably just fine but was thrilled to have her company. We had spent very little time together just the two of us, and despite the eight year difference in our ages, we had become really good friends over the years. I was getting so spoiled with everyone cooking dinners for me. They always tasted better when I did not cook them. Another part of my diet was increasing my fruit and vegetable intake. Janet went to the grocery store to get healthy food, vegetables and fruit and proceeded to teach me to make smoothies and vegetable sandwiches. We had an early night because as always after chemotherapy I was really exhausted.

When I awakened, I was so happy and content. I thanked God because I realized again that He had been answering my prayers all along, including those I couldn't or didn't dare to speak; like would I survive surgery and chemotherapy or would this cancer kill me. As I remembered the last months, I realized that I have more answered prayers than I can even begin to count. Each passing day had taught me something else about myself or my faith or my God or my love for my family and friends.

Janet set out that day to fill me with more healthy food than any ten people could eat, and I did learn how to make an amazing smoothie with about 4-5 servings of fruit. That's more than half of the total I need in a day. The fruit smoothie became a staple of my diet and I had one for lunch daily. There's no refined sugar in them. From all that I read refined sugar was the enemy and it would be eliminated. I tried to increase my intake of complex carbohydrates. Jim, Justin, and Kate arrived home from Orlando that day and Janet cooked dinner for the whole family. Years ago she made a meal called 'crazy mixed up crust something' so she decided to improve on it and make it healthy. It was absolutely the worst! Sometimes things should stay unhealthy. She thought it was awful too, but we all ate it.

She was leaving the next morning and it was hard to say goodbye particularly since her Army Reserve Unit was potentially going to get called up to go to the Middle East. I won't worry about this because worry was senseless. I was learning. I knew God was there, and always had been, but I have been a senseless worrier forever. Janet left among laughter and tears and I immersed myself in the scrapbooks to help the time pass. I continued all my other interests too and I was feeling really good. I even managed to quit taking sleeping pills every night. It was not a problem at all, despite having taken them regularly for the last six months. Now I only needed one occasionally. This was progress, and I did not become addicted as I feared might happen.

As was the typical pattern for the day after chemotherapy, I had the worst metallic taste in my mouth thanks to the controlled poisoning. I noticed it but I could still eat so it was just a minor nuisance. Food tasted strange. But this was the last time I would have the taste.

Now all along I expected my eyebrows and eyelashes to fall out and they had not. I had no hair on my head. I had little hair on my arms and legs. My pubic hair was gone. I kept thinking if I was just really gentle and careful, the hair around my eyes would stay. The last and final blow to my body image began happening about ten days after the final chemo, when my eyebrows started to get that funny itchy feeling that my scalp had done previously. Within a few days, my eyebrows were gone. Not entirely, but what was left was so blond you could barely see that I even had eyebrows. I tried eye brow pencil and it was a disaster. I looked like a poorly painted porcelain doll. I decided a few blond brows were sufficient and would have to do. Then the eyelashes started to fall out. Lash by lash they fell like leaves falling from the trees in early autumn. Within days, I was left with forty percent of my original eyelashes. Now I began to painstakingly put makeup on every day. I would carefully put on a lash thickener and mascara lash by lash and it looked pretty good if I had to say so myself. I only had to survive this humiliation briefly because much to my joy, the eyebrows and lashes started to come back very quickly. Within a month many had satisfactorily returned, so I felt much better. Last to fall out and first to grow back. I had no idea.

I still meditated and prayed and exercised and read my Bible everyday. I took regular rest periods and stretched out with a dog on either side of me. Our dogs were such good and faithful friends throughout my whole ordeal and they were not about to leave me now. They seemed to sense something because they had not been out of my sight much for months.

I decided that I would get into a Bible study of some type after this ordeal. There was a lot of peace in the Bible reading that I was doing right now but it was pretty unorganized. I opened my bible and started to read wherever it happened to be on any given day. I needed to keep my brain stimulated and my thoughts on God and recovery.

I was getting closer to my follow up appointment one month after the end of chemotherapy with the oncologist. I still felt strong and was able to exercise more each day. My friends were still hanging in there, but thankfully, my needs were far less. Geri came down almost every weekend and that was something for me to look forward to. Jim's and my intimacy returned to normal or maybe even a little better. He was still afraid of crushing my breasts and rupturing the implants. We would get more comfortable with this I am sure. I was not ready to discuss this with any of the doctors and hopefully would not have to. Generally I was pretty open but there was a limit to my candidness. You would think I would have gotten rid of my prudish behavior years ago.

On Sunday, the 16th of February, I went to church for the first time since October. I really missed going. I hoped that my immune system was strong and could fight off any germs that would be lurking. Again I felt pretty self conscious because very few people knew what had happened and I wore my wig. Although it looked similar to what my own hair used to be, it looked different enough for people to notice. At least I thought they noticed. I sat in the middle of the family since I was not sure about my immune system, and if I sat on an end I had to hold hands with other people and have more contact with those around me. It was great to be back and doing something normal. It had been a very long time since anything was normal. It was good to get used to wearing my wig in public since I still would not have hair for quite awhile.

The following day was Monday, and I saw the oncologist for my first post chemotherapy visit and I felt great. I had not had a menstrual period and I thought that was a good sign. I kept hoping that I was already menopausal, since I erroneously thought somehow I would not need the tamoxifen if I were. I had enough symptoms and hot flashes that I would not notice a difference when I started on the tamoxifen, which was necessary. The oncologist was happy with my recovery although my immune system was still compromised. I was afraid that would impact the removal of my port in three days but he did not think so. I was relieved. I wanted the port out most of all. I had no unusual lumps or bumps or lymph nodes. I didn't think I could hear that enough. He told me to go ahead and start the tamoxifen tonight. I would be taking it twice a day. We reviewed the side effects again and he told me to feel free to call if I needed to. The anticipation of this was almost worse than the chemotherapy, but not quite. I left the office happy to be alive and ready to embark on my further adventures with breast cancer. I waited until later to take the first tamoxifen. It was a little like anticipating the birth of a baby. Once the baby was born you could not turn around and put it back in. Once I had taken the first tamoxifen there was no turning back and I certainly wouldn't want to, considering the benefit of this drug in estrogen receptor positive tumors. I so desperately wanted survival. Certainly, as a nurse going through this, the experience would help me deal with others who may be facing the same diagnosis. You can always teach better if you've experienced what you are teaching. I managed to get through the first few days of tamoxifen and so far so good. The hot flashes were the only real problem. I had not experienced the extent of the hot flashes associated with menopause and tamoxifen together. I waited to get through the first month which was supposedly the worst.

As the month progressed, I realized that I did not become instantly psychotic and I did not threaten my husband's life, even once. Since I was most likely menopausal, the fears that come each year as that transition grew closer for my age group, was a nonissue for me. I found that to be a relief as well as never having to deal with the hormone replacement debate. I talked to a pharmacist at an integrative pharmacy to see if there was anything I should be taking that I was not. He suggested only the addition of Omega 3 Fatty Acid Oil Capsules. I definitely decided to do that, especially when he said it would put more moisture in my skin and keep it softer.

One of the problems with menopause was the dryness of everything.

I would be remiss if I did not discuss the truth about hot flashes. I won't dismiss the fact that they were not the most pleasant experience. However, they were not as bad as I expected, and I reasoned that I could put up with a lot with the knowledge that it increased the likelihood of survival. I got hot flashes all day and all night. During the day they posed a few more problems because I always seemed to get them when I was trying to put on makeup and the makeup would not stick to my sweaty face. I forged ahead and did the best that I could, and depending on who might be around at the time, could often just joke about them. I considered it a nice sweaty glow. I was very open about hot flashes too. Jim thought too much so but again I thought I could use the experience to educate women. The key to hot flash survival I found was 'lukewarm'. I used to think lukewarm was wishy washy, but if I kept everything lukewarm I was much more comfortable. I ate lukewarm soup. I drank lukewarm liquids. I made my green tea and let it sit for twenty minutes and then drank it. I took lukewarm baths and showers. Extremes in temperature tended to make the hot flashes occur with more frequency. I had two fans going in my room on either side of the bed. I used to awaken with each hot flash, now I only got up once with the 2:00 am hot flash. Yes, I had one every night around that time. I could almost set an alarm. I got up and usually got a drink of water, sat in front of the fan briefly and then lay down on top of my covers. The fans blew directly on me. I used the time I was awake to pray about things I forgot to pray about during the day since I had no distractions at that hour. Eventually, I cooled off enough to the point I began to freeze, and then I got back under the covers and fell back asleep. During the rest of the night, I almost subconsciously was able to push off all the covers and then put them all back on as the hot flashes came and went. I never traveled without my fan. I used to wake up soaking wet and shivering but the fan helped me dry out so to speak. Initially I ran to the mirror every time I had a hot flash to see what I looked like. I realized that I didn't turn beet red and probably no one could tell, although my face did glow. The perspiration was not dripping down my face and body although it sure felt like it was. I did start to itch all over with extreme hot flashes. I do not discount that some people may have really severe hot flashes but as annoying as mine seemed, they were tolerable. Along with the hot flashes I also had a great deal of trouble with temperature regulation. I had solved that dilemma and carried around half my wardrobe at all times. I learned that cotton was an indispensable fabric. It's absorbent and dried quickly. I was surviving the hot flashes with cotton clothing that I wore in layers and always had more clothes than I needed for any event because I could count on being both very hot and very cold.

Chapter 14

Subsequent Surgeries

I scheduled port removal on February 20th, a few days after I saw the oncologist. This day could not come soon enough. I believed the port had been the most annoying thing to deal with. It was a constant reminder that you had cancer and were getting chemotherapy. Mine just always seemed to be in the way. It rubbed everything, all the time.

Once again because of the medicine they liked to administer during the procedure, I could not eat after midnight. I took my morning medicine with a few sips of water. I had to wait the whole morning because the surgery was at 12:30 pm again. This was the first time I had seen most of the staff since my mastectomy and reconstruction for the breast cancer, but this was pretty exciting. Finally, I didn't feel like the poster child of doom and gloom. I no longer felt as though everyone pitied me. They had a hard time starting my IV, which was unusual but having four months of chemotherapy tended to trash your veins. I also only had one arm that could be used because of the lymph node dissection on the left side. After several tries I had an IV and I was ready to go. It was still freezing in the OR but I could care less. The port was coming out and I had looked forward to this day since the day it had been placed in November.

I think I slept through most of the procedure because I don't remember being as chatty as I would normally be with the conscious sedation. Some scar tissue had grown around the port just as it does around my implants because it was a foreign object under my skin. The general surgeon removed that as well, so I wouldn't have a lump of scar tissue under the skin on my chest. She was finally done and I went to the recovery area where I got some crackers and juice and was home before the kids got home from school at 3:00. I always slept a lot during the days after each episode of sedation.

I got in a few naps but Kate had her first dance competition in two days and I must take her to a dress rehearsal and to downtown Denver for the competition. The day of the actual competition was fairly long and tiring and a little hard but she and I both made it through the day. This was one of the first times other than church that I had been out in a crowd with my wig so I felt a little conspicuous. Since it was winter I wore warm hats a lot so the wig took some getting used to, particularly wearing it eight to ten hours straight. Every cough I heard made me nervous as I tried to avoid all the sickness. It was still February and I thought the entire world had a cold.

I was an absolute fanatic about hand washing and keeping my family healthy. No one was allowed to enter the house sick, and everyone who came in washed their hands immediately, including all the kid's friends. During my nadir week I tried not to have kids in at all except my own. I carried antibacterial wipes in my car so anyone who got in the car had to wipe their hands, too. My family had to wash their hands whenever they came in the house, including my dad and every time someone sneezed or coughed they had to wash their hands again as well as when they were going to handle food. My feeling was that we could not be too careful. I had become the queen of hand washing but it was a terrific habit to get into and I hoped it continued. As a result of this vigilance I had not been sick since before my surgery and I was so thankful. The common cold was anything but common when your immune system was being tortured and destroyed. Some have survived chemotherapy only to die of pneumonia or some other secondary infection.

I felt like a butterfly emerging from a cocoon. I missed the sense of accomplishment I got from completing scrapbook pages, but it was great to be alive and start simple things like carpooling and grocery shopping. My wig was a permanent part of me now. I didn't notice it as much and I didn't feel like it screamed wig when I was out. Kate had another dance competition in another few weeks. Baseball was starting and the High School team was planning a trip for Spring Break. They were driving to Arizona and at first I thought I could drive it all myself with Ryan. It seemed like a vacation in warm weather could be nice. However during the planning process I realized that the trip would be too much this soon after treatment and I would enjoy being home when Jerred came home for his Spring Break. I had grandiose ideas but reality fortunately prevailed. I got very tired very quickly and had to lie down right away when it hit me.

It had been 6 months since my breast cancer diagnosis was made. I had several more follow-up appointments. I started to consider the surgery to reconstruct nipples and areola that would complete the reconstructive process. I was so happy to be done with the original surgery and chemotherapy that I could finally look toward the future. This was something I had been afraid to do before now. I felt very buxom, but, I was actually only a C cup. Having been a AA, it was a pretty drastic change for me. I was getting used to having breasts and was glad I made the decision I had. I would not have liked to have the mastectomy without the reconstruction, but I'm sure I would have adjusted. Not everyone was lucky enough to be able to do both at the same time, and I had a great result because of the ability to combine the two surgeries. God continued to answer my prayers guiding me in all my decisions. Finally the breasts were becoming part of me and not just two foreign objects plopped on my chest. Calling them my breasts was a stretch, and would still take some time.

March brought a little more normalcy to our lives. Although I checked daily there was not much hair on my head. Amazingly, pubic, leg, and arm hair had all returned, although less than previous amounts. I started to think about things other than cancer. It had consumed every waking moment for the past six months.

I realized that I needed to write thank you notes to everyone who had done something thoughtful over the past six months. It would take hours of my time and I still could not possibly begin to express my gratitude so I started to plan a 'thank you' party with a caterer. The caterer was great because she took my feelings and emotions and suggested different ideas that were suitable. I first decided that I would have an early evening Open House since bedtime was about seven o'clock each evening and even then I was totally exhausted. I wanted the party to be festive with bright spring colors and good food and plenty of drinks for everyone. I also wanted a lot of flowers all over the house since it was spring and a time of rebirth. I felt as though it was my rebirth. The human spirit was resilient. As I tried to set a date, I realized that there was only one Saturday that would work for months and that was the 12th of April and so that was the date. I was so excited to be able to do this and it was something fun to plan between soccer, baseball games, and track meets. My sister, who was indeed mobilized with her Army Reserve Unit to go to Turkey, was at Ft Hood, Texas in a holding pattern waiting to find out when she would be leaving. She got some time off and flew in for the party and Geri came down from Ft Collins. Even my dad rallied and wanted to come for as long as possible. My niece and nephew and their kids planned to come as well. My extended family was well represented as they too were continually impressed with and wanted to thank my friends as well.

This was the first big party I had given, and my only fear was that I had bitten off more than I could chew so soon after my treatments had ended. As it turned out, the party was a huge success. It exceeded my expectations and gave me a chance to thank friends and family personally. Even those who were unable to attend, I was able to thank when they called to RSVP. I have saved all the notes and cards I received over the months so that I could look back at them and maybe put together some kind of a memory book. I really did not want to ever forget this whole experience and its highs and lows. Every minute, no matter how hard, had given me such new perspectives on the world and my life.

This summer was my 30 year high school reunion. I had not heard anything about it for so long that I thought that nothing was planned. I had no hair and I didn't even know if I wanted to go back to Rapid City, South Dakota. It turned out, however, that there was indeed a reunion planned for July and I tentatively agreed to go. I had a lot of misgivings. I felt like I was in contact with everyone I cared to be in contact with. It would be nice to go back since it's been five or six years since I had been there.

Also in the plans was a trip to a national dance competition with Kate, which included all the competitive dance teams at her studio. The competition was in Las Vegas, Nevada. I knew that if she was going to go, I would have to take her. This was not a dad and daughter event. We found that out at the Christmas recital when I was unable to attend and Jim and all dads were kicked out of the dressing room. He really was not much help trying to help Kate get dressed and get her hair and make up done prior to performances. I asked Geri if she would like to go with us. I knew I could not make the trip alone. I needed to drive and hoped to be able to sight see along the way. Geri loved Las Vegas so it didn't take much to convince her. I was thrilled to have the company. I was afraid to do anything by myself, and I knew that my white blood cell count was still not as high as I would have liked it to be. It seemed to be taking a really long time to bounce back. It sure didn't take as long to destroy my immune system with the controlled poisoning. Summer plans were started to materialize and it was great to move forward.

I had another appointment with the plastic surgeon and one of the breasts had significant scar tissue formed around the implant and had pushed a small bubble out the top that felt a little like a hernia. It was a little uncomfortable, too. It rubbed on my chest from the inside and caused irritation. As I planned for the nipple reconstruction, I also planned to have an open capsulotomy on the right side. That meant that the plastic surgeon would cut just under the right breast and actually go in and cut the scar in several places allowing the breast to fall back into the correct position and get rid of the little out pouching. This was very common with implants and I was not overly concerned. Unfortunately it required another round of conscious sedation and an operating room visit. Of course I could again have nothing to eat after midnight. I hated that part. No date was set but it would be soon.

About this time I started to get strange shooting pains around my back and up and down the mid-axillary lines under both arms. It felt a little like getting feeling back in your foot after it had fallen asleep. The pains were uncomfortable at times as they came in waves. The pain would shoot in and catch me by surprise and then would continue for a few hours to a day or so. These were actually normal and indicated that I was getting some sensation back in those areas. I knew I wouldn't have full sensation particularly under my left arm due to the lymph node dissection, but the return of sensation was nice to have since many areas of my back and sides had been numb since surgery.

I also began to notice that one or the other of the breasts would start to itch or have pain. The common reaction was to scratch or rub the area which I did only to be quickly reminded that I had two insensate breasts. I experienced phantom discomfort just like someone who had lost an arm or a leg and yet feels pain in the missing limb. The nerves still tell the brain that the missing part was present, even though it was not. At that point it was not serious. I knew however that it could become so painful and debilitating that it might require significant analgesia (pain relief).

I scheduled my next reconstructive procedure for the middle of May just after the end of the baseball, soccer, and track seasons. Each time I went into the outpatient surgery department I felt like the whole world knew I was there. Going in for my open capsulotomy and nipple construction was no different. I wondered if they were getting sick of seeing me. The nice thing was that I felt healthy and not frightened anymore. After all, the plastic surgeon was the fun doctor. She was not trying to poison me and never had bad news to give me. This was a minor procedure. I don't love being in the hospital and now the facility was in the middle of a huge remodeling project, so nothing was where it should be. For the first time I actually was scheduled in the morning. Although I had to be there at 6:30 am, I was glad to be going to surgery at 8:00 am. I received conscious sedation after they got the intravenous line running, which again was difficult because my veins were still scrawny from chemotherapy. It was still cold but I do not think that will ever change. I was wearing a hat and they allowed me to keep it on to stay warm and I just put the surgical cap over it. That helped a lot in keeping warm since 95% of our body heat escaped through the head. I arrived in the operating room and was fairly awake. I wanted to know what was happening. The open capsulotomy was first and it seemed to take forever. I knew that I was awake because I kept asking the plastic surgeon questions. Apparently I kept asking her if she had a significant other. It seemed like a reasonable question but I asked it four or five times and it became fairly humorous for everyone except me because I forgot I asked the question and could not remember the answer. I felt pressure, but no pain but I heard the scissors cutting the scar tissue. The sensation was odd. I remembered her completing the capsulotomy and telling me that she was starting to form the nipples. I got a little groggier so I don't remember much after that until she started to stitch the nipples. She was able to form them using the skin on the breast mound. I was afraid they would use labia tissue or groin tissue as they had in the past and that seemed far too barbaric. I was so reassured to find out they would use breast skin and not a skin graft. The surgery went quickly now and I was rolled into the recovery area. The whole procedure had taken three hours and I was amazed that it had been that long.

I seemed to be whisked out of the hospital really fast compared to the other times and I was very sleepy. I think I ate when I got home and could not get into bed fast enough. My window cleaner was at the house and he came into the bedroom to clean the inside of the windows and I hardly noticed. I just told him to go ahead and not mind me sleeping on the bed. I slept for three hours. I cannot take the bandages off for another day and this time I was excited to see the results.

I had reason to be excited because when the bandages came off I had nipples and no longer an out pouching that looked like a hernia. The right breast had moved back down into place and looked more normal. I was thrilled and looked forward to getting the tattoo for the areola and nipple which could not be done for three weeks, until the newly operated on areas had healed.

Finally after waiting six months I made an appointment with my new primary care doctor for a much needed physical exam. I had put off having a repeat Pap smear for many months longer that I should have but I did so at the request of my oncologist who did not think I needed to deal with any more health issues. I was sure he believed that getting any more bad news would have devastated me. I had lab work drawn and went over all my medications and the list was really growing now. I felt so old because I had to type up the medication list and carry it in my wallet so I would not forget what I was taking, just like all the old people I knew. The doctor and I discussed my need to have a heel densitometry done to screen for bone mass changes. Heel densitometry was a very easy, painless screening to assess bone density. One thing I remembered from all the dinner lectures Jim and I attended was the necessity for a baseline bone density at the time of menopause. I was pronounced as healthy as I could be under the circumstances. Luckily all my blood work was normal except my white blood cells and granulocytes, which are still low four months after the last chemotherapy. My Pap smear was absolutely normal. I breathed a little sigh of relief. Something else was normal. I value normal more and more. It was great to be among the majority.

I had an appointment to see the oncologist about that time too, which always made my anxiety level rise. It was only a routine follow-up appointment. I already knew my lab values were within normal limits so there was little he could find that I did not already know. I was really excited to show off my new nipples. He even took off the bandages so he could see them. He completed an exam and there was nothing new and I felt good. My white count was still low and my immune system was not back to normal. So it was taking me a little longer to get it back. I'm sure this was not unusual. I actually had no idea but rationalized many things now.

I received permission from the plastic surgeon and the oncologist to run in The Bolder Boulder which is a 10 kilometer race that was one of the top races of its kind in the nation. I ran a quarter of a mile training run to prepare for it. This was pathetic after the training I had done for other races in my life but it was the best I could do. The Saturday night before the race, as I was sitting in bed watching television, I decided that I would perform a self-breast exam. My heart stopped momentarily as I felt another suspicious lump on the right breast fairly laterally but concerning none the less. I was immediately transported back to the day I found the first lump the previous September. I mourned my mother all over again and felt that same deep despair and devastation. It felt exactly as the other lump had felt and I even made Geri feel it so she would have the experience of feeling a breast lump. I was not going to leave her out of this learning process. Not everyone knows what they are feeling for. I showed it to Jim and made him feel it. He did not seem too concerned but I knew I needed to follow up and it was Memorial Day weekend so nothing would be open until Tuesday. I tried hard not to think about it and prayed that it would not be cancer again. The one thing I remembered the general surgeon telling me was that if I had a recurrence it would be superficial and easy to find.

I made it through the weekend and the race and ran almost the whole distance because my six year old sprinted the whole way or she stopped and rode on her father's shoulders. I bet she ran at least half the distance. I realized, early on in the race that I could not sprint to keep up with her and tried to keep a steady pace while Jim kept up with Kate. The race was so much fun and I thought the miles passed very quickly. I could not believe we were really at Folsum Field, the Football Stadium at the University of Colorado and the race was over. Our time was one hour and twenty-four minutes, not a great time, but it was one of the biggest victories in my life. I haven't run a race in twenty two years and I ran this one after chemotherapy. What a thrill the moment I started to run into the stadium for the last lap. Since I was at the end of the racers, the stadium was full of cheering fans. It took my breath away. This was such a personal victory for me. No one else had any idea but me. I felt as if I just won the race of my life and in a matter of speaking I had. I survived breast cancer, major surgery, and chemotherapy. This race was not unlike the journey I had taken through this past 9 months. As hard as I tried not to think about it, that new lump was a bit distracting.

On Tuesday morning I called my surgeon and she was out of town. I called my husband to see if my primary care physician would remove the lump but he said no because it was too close to the implant so I called my new best friend, the plastic surgeon. I felt desperate but I got an appointment, finally. It was late in the afternoon but I did not really care because someone was going to feel the lump and take it out immediately. I worried all day because it felt just like the lump I had felt previously that had been diagnosed as cancer even though no one thought it was cancer. I think I had become permanently skeptical. I tried to pray away my anxiety. Surely, God would not let it happen to me again. I knew for sure that He would not abandon me now. It definitely helped but I was still quite concerned and knew I wanted to have this lump removed right away. My general surgeon had told me when I asked her how to perform self-breast exams after the mastectomy to check from just under the breast to the neck and from mid axillary line to mid axillary line and include under the arms.

This lump was just along the mid-axillary line on the right side. I arrived at my appointment and was escorted into the exam room. I felt that I looked visibly shaken, and I am sure it seemed fairly obvious. The plastic surgeon, with a little worry on her face, felt the lump and although not sure about it said we could schedule the operating room and remove it. I did not want to wait for that and prevailed upon her to take it out immediately. I don't even know if she removed lumps and bumps as we liked to call them, but I was not going home until this lump was gone. I actually helped her remove it so she did not need to call her medical assistant. When she showed it to me, it looked like a lymph node but I had been deceived before so I really would not relax until the pathology report came back. It would take ten days to two weeks. I went home feeling much better since the lump was gone but still a little worried about what it might be. I could not rush anything so I had to be content with just waiting.

This was a very busy time of the year with the end of the school year coming in the next week and I threw myself into this to forget the waiting. I volunteered to help with Kate's Kindergarten graduation since it would be quite a festive event. Every milestone in grade school was a continuation event and thus worthy of celebration. We lived in a very touchy, feely school district. All the children and teachers must feel good about themselves all the time. Everything that I did became so much more meaningful to me since I was so thankful to be here. I had undergone such tremendous personal and physical changes. Every color seemed more vivid this spring and every event more important and fun.

Finally about eight days later the pathology results were in and the plastic surgeon called to tell me that the lump was indeed just a lymph node with no evidence of metastatic disease. Wow, those words were music to my ears. She could have become one of the *not fun* doctors quickly, with different results. It was anyone's guess how it got where it was on my body but I had a complicated surgery and the reconstruction involved a lot of tissue being moved around. I was so relieved. I had gotten another result that was absolutely normal. It was so nice to be normal. It had been a long time since anything regarding my breasts had been normal. The most frightening aspect was that everything had always looked normal. I had the plastic surgeon fax me the results too since I needed to read the absolute proof and see the results myself. Medical science had let me down too many times recently when things looked normal.

My hair had been slowly growing in and I had what looked like blond goose down all over my head. This was a far cry from the gray hair my husband Jim thought was coming in a month ago. Of course I examined it quite carefully every day to see if it was growing. It seemed to be growing so slowly but when you consider that it had to grow from the follicle and that was located well under the scalp, it took time for the hair to just reach the surface of the scalp. It's not quite like just shaving your head and then growing your hair out. I needed to keep reminding myself of this since I was really anxious to have my hair back. I wore baseball caps now instead of the wig and I felt very comfortable. The weather was getting warm and the wig just got too hot especially when I was dealing with hot flashes as well. I was worried that I wouldn't have hair for my 30th High School reunion in July and I was thinking I might not go. I had beautiful long blond hair all through school. I knew that was still what people expected to see, not to mention I weighed 25 pounds less than I did when I graduated from high school. I had registered to attend but I was having second thoughts. I looked a little like a walking skeleton. There is an unrealistic and strange perception before reunions that we expect everyone to look as we had thirty years before. Obviously, very few people did.

Kate's graduation from kindergarten was great fun and there were lots of tears. The cakes were unique because each cake had an enlarged picture of each class on it that was actually part of the frosting and was edible. This was my last child to leave kindergarten and I was entitled to shed a few tears. I was so glad I did not have to deal with any other graduations this year. I still cried at the drop of a hat and was so emotional. Much of that emotion is just the extraordinary joy I feel each day when I wake up and count my blessings. I never wanted to lose the ability to feel that. It almost made the difficult events of the past year tolerable. Next year we would have an eighth grader and a senior who would both graduate, and that was soon enough for another round of continuation events.

Finally three weeks after my nipple surgery, I was ready for the final step. The plastic surgeon would tattoo the nipples and areola on both breasts. Again, she wanted to do the procedure in the operating room but I could not face that place again, so I persuaded her to perform the procedure in the office where all the equipment was located. This whole debate goes on because sometimes the insurance company in its infinite wisdom will not pay her to do the tattooing in the office for about one tenth of the cost of the hospital outpatient surgery department. This caused me to wonder how many other stupid decisions were made by insurance companies thus increasing the cost of premiums for no good reason. I had already experienced a few. I had no feeling in my breasts so there would be no need for any anesthesia, which would be a reason to have the procedure done in the hospital. I shuddered to think of the awful places that some people choose to get their tattoos. I had a few dreams in which I was getting my tattoo at some tattoo parlor called 'Tiny's'. The place was filled with cigarette smoke and the smell of cheap booze and Tiny, at about 6 foot 5 inches tall and 300 pounds, was the tattoo artist. I had lived near or on many military installations each with their own *strips* with bars, pawn shops, and tattoo parlors lining the streets directly outside the post. We finally compromised and decided to try the procedure in the office. Again I do not even know if there was an insurance code for the procedure so that it could be charged to the insurance company but it was all part of the reconstruction.

I was a little nervous having never gotten a tattoo before, but the process was pretty simple. It involved an electric handle with several needles attached that picked up the dye and then made small pin pricks in the skin where the nipples had been reconstructed, in the area where the areola should be. The dye was then embedded in those areas. It was a little noisy but I only felt a little pressure. The plastic surgeon freehanded the tattoo meaning there was no drawing or stencil to mark where the tattoo would be. I was so impressed, and I marveled at how artistically gifted she was to be to be able to do such fine work. I was reminded of the great artists who created life sized sculptures, like Michelangelo and his David. I envisioned that she had talent something like that. Upon completion, the nipples looked dark but she assured me that they would lighten over time. It was better to start with them dark because as they began to lighten, I would not have to get the tattoos repeated. Of course the sites were bandaged and I would not see her for follow-up until after I returned from Las Vegas. I could remove the bandages after 24 hours.

I tried to plan the trip to Las Vegas for Kate's dance competition and my *lemon* of a van had finally pushed me over the edge. The sliding door never did work quite right and did not close fifty percent of the time. I started looking at new cars, and concurrently Jim had been looking for a new car for himself too. We actually settled on buying two new cars and I picked up a new van the day before Geri, Kate, and I were scheduled to leave for Las Vegas. All these little stressors that would have been a tremendous annoyance to me in the past seemed to have little effect on my spirits. I was able to take the car buying in stride. Normally a purchase of that magnitude would have kept me awake for several nights. Things just happen and not always at the best time. Certainly my breast cancer didn't come at a good time, but then when is there ever a good time to find out that you have any cancer?

We managed an early start for the trip to Las Vegas and the first day we arrived with enough time to visit Bryce Canyon National Park in Utah. It was a long, hot drive but the new car was much more comfortable and smooth riding than the old one and it had an entertainment center so Kate could watch movies and play games. We only had to figure out how it worked. Geri became a pro. We entered Bryce Canyon about five in the afternoon. At first it looked like there was nothing there, but then as we rounded a bend in the road, as if out of nowhere, a breathtaking canyon filled with late afternoon shadows and beautiful colors appeared. Just being there sharing this with my daughter and her Godmother Geri was another answer to prayer for me. There were many times along the journey the past year when I did not think I would figuratively get around all the bends in the road to see such beauty again. The vastness of the scenery and the millions of years it took to form this canyon were awe inspiring. There were not as many people here as in other national parks so it was very enjoyable and we were able to see the entire canyon before dark.

On this trip, it became obvious that my hair was not growing back to look like it had been before the chemotherapy. At first it resembled an asparagus patch with strange little shoots of hair sticking straight up all by themselves. It also seemed like it might be coming in gray, but then it appeared possibly blond or light brown. I could now shampoo and rinse. There was actually something on my head to wash, even though I never quit shampooing during the past many months with no hair. As for the color, I decided that I would highlight it before the reunion so I was not too concerned. If indeed it was coming in a darker color than I was used to, there was always hair color which would allow me to gently ease into my new hair. What was taking some getting used to was the fact that it was very curly. In fact, 'Curly' had become my new nickname. I'm now five months out from chemotherapy and still had very little hair but enough so that I got by with no hat or just a baseball cap. The baseball cap was more to protect my head from sunburn than cover my head because of no hair. I had never had curly hair and this was looking quite different and only time would tell, but right now it sure was easy to take care of. I called it my 'wash and wear' hair. My eyelashes and eyebrows were thickening more. I found that the loss of this hair was the most difficult to accept, after the pubic hair, of course.

We hustled on the way home from Las Vegas, because Ryan had a baseball tournament and I wanted to try to see a game. Also, if we made it home in time on the fourth of July, I would be able to go to our annual neighborhood block party. The trip home was uneventful and we made it in plenty of time for a game and the party. The fireworks were more spectacular than ever. However, standing for long periods of time was difficult since my back would get sore. I still felt really tight around my chest. In fact, it felt like a large rubber band was around my chest. I had added some physical therapy exercises to my normal workout in an attempt to stay loose but the tightness lingered.

I was nine months out from surgery but my pectoralis major muscles, which are the muscles across the front of each side of the chest, were still very tight since the implants were placed under them. Stretching on my foam roll was great therapy and felt pretty good. My back was tight from the incisions. My biggest problem seemed to be that I just did not have enough skin to go around and so when incisions were sutured, they were just tight. I worked on stretching everything out and hoped I would still get a bit looser and more comfortable in time. I also had a tendency to hunch my shoulders and I did not know why that was, but I was sure it had something to do with the fact that the pectoralis muscles along the upper chest were big and strong and without latissimus dorsi muscles I had to train new muscles to counter *the pull of the pecs*. I was still happy with the decision to have this type of reconstruction despite the minor inconveniences and discomfort. That's not to say that it didn't take determination to get used to it.

I was so at peace with all the decisions I had made. I really believed that God helped me make all the right decisions along the journey. I was reminded of a poem called Footprints. God walks along with us as evidenced by two sets of footprints, and then suddenly only one set of footprints is visible when the going becomes rough and treacherous, and the writer wonders what happened. Feeling abandoned, he asks where God was when the going got so hard. The answer of course, was that during those difficult times, God lifted him up and carried him. That is an image I will always hold onto. My faith continued to grow stronger as I looked back at the events of the past year and ahead to the future. I had to deal with my own mortality and grieved for the loss of body parts. I grieved the loss of many other things, not the least of whom was my mother, my best friend. Without God helping me over each of these hurdles, in addition to just keeping a family as large as mine functioning, I thought I would surely have jumped off a tall building by now. Prayer helped me sort out what was really important and what was not. I knew that the answers would come, maybe not in the time frame I would have liked, but I trusted they would come. I had felt the presence of God and I wanted to make sure that I did not lose this close spiritual relationship. I received a gift when I started this adventure with cancer. I wanted to commit to memory every single event that had occurred. This diagnosis could well be, in an odd sort of way, the best thing that had ever happened to me. Only time would tell.

Part 3

Chapter 15

The True Test

As I prepared for my next trip I was very apprehensive. Returning to Rapid City as a cancer survivor scared me. I had changed. This was the place of my youth when we didn't have to worry about the bad things in life. My life there had been happy and carefree. One thing I wanted to do was go fishing because the thought of sitting on a boat in the cool morning waiting for the fish to bite sounded blissfully relaxing. Having never been much of a fisherman this struck me as odd, but Geri and her mom and dad arranged for all of us to get a pontoon boat and go fishing at Lake Pactola. I spent time there when I was a teenager but most of that time was spent water skiing or picnicking. This would be a new experience and I was looking forward to the relaxation.

I had a terrible time trying to pack and figure out what I needed and what I was still able to wear that was flattering and did not accentuate my short hair or my significant weight loss. This was just vanity and I had a few stern words with myself as well and said a few prayers to take this nonsense out of my head. I managed to get everything together and get off about ten in the morning. I wanted to be there by happy hour and in time to see a band concert.

I had been part of the Rapid City Municipal Band when I was in High School and during the summer they played weekly concerts in the park. It was a bit of lasting Americana. One of the people I respected most in my life was my band director. The lessons he taught me have continued to impact my life ever since my youth. He taught me to never be happy with giving 100% when I could give 110%. The other thought he etched into my brain was the saying; "Results, not excuses." Striving for excellence had become such a part of my life in the army, raising my children, and battling cancer.

My trip to South Dakota was beautiful and as I listened to music on the way my mind just drifted through so many thoughts. I rejoiced in the Lord through Christian music. I had time to pray about so many things. I also had time to shed a few tears because this was the first time I have ever gone to Rapid City and not had my mother there waiting to greet me. It was also not my home anymore. I guess I was grieving the loss of the innocence of youth too. I did not have any idea what to expect at this reunion but I sure was looking forward to it now. It was one of many tests of my survival. I would have to admit the cancer since I cannot hide my very curly short hair. I did not want to hide it either because if I could touch one life and encourage women in their self-breast exams, mammography, and annual physical exams, I would feel like I had truly made a difference. The concert was terrific and we ran into a few classmates there. It was quite a walk down memory lane because many songs they played were songs we played years ago. The highlight was getting to see both my band director and his wife. We talked with them quite awhile after a major commotion died down. A girl passed out in the bathroom and someone came looking for a nurse and after looking around I realized that I'd better go assess the situation and make sure she was breathing and had a heart rate. Someone else called an ambulance so I could give the dispatcher some idea of what was going on. One of my classmates, Karen, who was carrying her poodle went to direct the emergency vehicles as they came in. Karen was a former Miss South Dakota and was very attractive. It was so funny to see her with the dog in the middle of the street trying to direct the emergency vehicles and move the civilian vehicles out of the way. It was hot and very humid and the little bathroom was stifling. The perspiration was running down my face as I was suspended between the stall walls bent over trying to keep myself from falling with a leg against each wall. My legs were getting sore so I could not wait for the paramedics to arrive and after what seemed like an eternity, I was happy to hand off the young woman to the paramedics. She seemed to be fine but I would not let her get up until the paramedics immobilized her neck. Of course by that time there were police, firemen, and the ambulance crew in attendance. It was all quite exciting and a real welcome back to reality, my life as a nurse, and my new reality.

We were finally able to go back to catching up with all our lives in the last thirty years and I shared my story with the band director and his wife. Amazingly his wife had just completed her second series of chemotherapy for ovarian cancer and their thirty four year old daughter was finishing chemotherapy for breast cancer. The prevalence of cancer was so astonishing and it never ceased to amaze me how many people were touched by it. I, of course explained that my hair was not always short and curly which they knew. I have been so consumed with my own trials I forgot that others struggle as well. We shared quite a common bond.

The fishing trip the next morning was wonderfully relaxing and I caught five trout that we planned to eat that night. Water was very rejuvenating and just floating around waiting for fish to bite was so calming. It was exactly what I needed before the excitement of the reunion.

We had lunch the following day at the Country Club with friends and ran into other friends who were just starting the back nine of the golf course as we arrived for lunch. These guys had been good friends but I did not recognize any of them. We went through mandatory hugs all around and as we walked in to take our seats, I turned to ask Geri who they all were. I was terribly embarrassed. It turned out that one of them was a guy I had dated for awhile and gone with to Prom and I didn't even recognize him. Of course it had been thirty years. We all had a great laugh and as it turned out he did not know who I was either and neither did any of the others because I looked so different. But it was OK. We had a wonderful lunch catching up on what everyone was doing and had been doing and then took golf carts out on the course to bother the guys again. I was astonished that anyone would let us take two golf carts anywhere. It was great to see them and we ended up spending a fair amount of time with them all. I started to feel better about coming because instead of feeling sorry for me, friends seem to be amazed at my resilience and courage. I had not thought of myself as resilient or courageous. It made me feel really good so that when I went to the cocktail party that night, I did not feel like I stood out. That neon sign on my forehead that blinked cancer for months was gone. I was different but not worried about what anyone thought. I had spent months worrying about this reunion and almost did not come for no good reason. It was such fun to be with all these friends. It was almost as if time stood still and we were back in High School again without any of the pressures of adolescence or growing up. I laughed so hard and most exciting, we got to do this all again the next night. I couldn't wait.

Geri committed to a golf game in the morning at nine and it was 1:30 in the morning before we got home. I did not have that kind of energy yet. More power to her. I don't play golf but a few friends and I decided we are going to learn before the next reunion which we may have sooner than later because of how well we all got along. I woke up about 10:00 am and ate quickly figuring the golfers would be making the turn at the tenth hole and sure enough they were so I took some great pictures. Although I was using my antiquated 35 mm camera it provided a great opportunity to get a group shot. We spent the rest of the day engaged in fun activities. I drove by my old house and my elementary school and through the neighborhood where I grew up. It looked so much the same and yet so different. Memories came flooding back into my mind and they were wonderful. All of these things had taken on such significance to me after the past year. I was so grateful to be here to do all this. I would not have missed this for the world. There was such joy and love. My family would not have enjoyed the trip and that was why they stayed home, but for the classmates it was wonderful. Even some of the spouses had a good time even though most left early, if they got a chance. These people had done well through the years and I liked who they chose to marry and I still liked them, some even more than I had in the past. It was so hard to see the night end but I had to leave by 10:00 am the next morning so I really needed to get some sleep. I still fatigued easily, and I really needed to get home to help Justin with a formal etiquette dinner he was planning for Monday night.

As hard as it was to leave, I said my good-byes and then my old friend Jim walked me to the car with Geri. He told me how courageous I was and how much he respected me and what I had been through. I was in tears of course as I always was these days. I would really miss everyone and I thought that I couldn't wait for the next reunion. It felt so good to finally think about five years from the present, as in five year survival. We actually decided to try to plan something in Colorado or Las Vegas before the next reunion, perhaps in the year we would all be turning fifty years old. At our twentieth reunion we decided not to meet for ten more years. This time we decided to get together before forty years, which I think is really terrific. I was so thrilled to learn that so many classmates were living in Colorado. I planned to see some of them when I went to Vail for Justin's soccer tournament in August.

My trip home was again one of reflection and prayer. I felt so good emotionally after a terrific weekend. I was so glad that God led me on this excursion. I made contact with so many people with whom I really do not want to lose contact again. Sharing my story of breast cancer was not difficult at all and not surprisingly, I found many others have suffered trials through their lives too. I was not quite sure why I thought these things only happened to me. We tend to think very egocentrically when we are ill.

I thought the experience of the reunion weekend reassured me that I actually could talk about the cancer, teach people something, and maybe even learn more myself. Perhaps I needed to find a way to get this story out. Thoughts of writing a book started during my drive back to Colorado. I wanted to use my experience with breast cancer to teach others and I wanted to share my journey of hope and prayer.

After getting home, I had a follow up appointment with the plastic surgeon to check the tattoos. They had healed beautifully and looked very normal. In fact, to look at me naked from a distance, you would have difficulty being able to tell that I even had the plastic surgery. It had exceeded my expectations.

I noticed while I was traveling that I had a something that looked very ropey extending from just under the left breast to my anterior superior iliac spine (pelvic bone). It felt like a cord and moved around when I pressed on it. I asked the plastic surgeon what it was and she had no idea. Now I decided I must have some sort of parasitic worm (helminth). It just moved up and down my abdomen. I set out to solve what in the world it might be. Thanks to John Link's book, <u>The Breast Cancer Survival Manual</u>, I decided that it was a clotted vein, which I rubbed, applied heat to and stretched until it slowly went away. I could not bring myself to see any more doctors for verification of my diagnosis.

Chapter 16

The Perfect Support Group

Many sources of information have encouraged me to find a support group to join. According to my alternative care doctor it actually helped in long term survival. Every time that I saw him or talked to him, he asked if I had found a group yet. This information proved to be elusive. Although I have found some support groups, they did not seem to be right for me. Some groups were for people with differing cancers and others seemed too morbid. Talking about death and dying was not something I wanted to do. I thought I could make it without one. Again I prayed that if one was out there that I could be part of that God would just drop it on my lap. Sure enough that's what happened.

I read in the newspaper one day about a group of cancer survivors who got together to hike, exercise, and swim. That sounded perfect. The group was called Rocky Mountain Team Survivor-Boulder. It took several days for me to contact the man who wrote the article and then several more days to contact the support group leader. I was not quite sure why this was so hard for me. I still felt emotionally raw and feared opening up to a group of strangers. Maybe I just feared that all a support group could offer me was an organized venue in which I can shed a lot of tears and ruminate over dying. Whatever caused me to drag my feet; I ultimately contacted the group leader after a bit of phone tag and started out with the weekly hike along Boulder Creek which was peaceful and serene. I was apprehensive about this experience. I met the group members slowly as they did not all come to hike every week, but we all shared our cancer stories over and over. In fact, that was the first thing we all did, when we met new people. At first it was hard to put the experience into words over and over, and of course I cried with each story. Amazingly, most of the women I shared with also began to cry. It seemed to be quite therapeutic. I kept thinking maybe I should not keep dwelling on it, but, I did not realize how much I needed this group until I started to meet them and share our experiences.

The time spent was very special and it introduced me to a whole new form of exercise, hiking. I learned about the trails in the area and which ones were good to take the whole family on including the dogs. In my short time with this group I felt as though I had good friends that share a very special bond. We were cancer survivors.

We cried together and rejoiced together. We ranged in age from 30 to 80. We had some women still in chemotherapy and others who were from a few months to 17 year survivors. We all understood the fragility of life and found joy in every single day. We shared problems and solutions and were very positive about our futures. I knew these women would continue to give me guidance for many years. I was not sure now why I had been so hesitant to find a group. I actually contemplated attending another support group for just breast cancer survivors but for now I was very happy with the group I had found.

The support group, as it turned out became a great place to share ups and downs and yes even commiserate over some of the side effects of different treatments. We bounced ideas off each other. It was a safe and nonjudgmental group that shared a common experience and talking about that experience. Talking about that experience was helpful in compartmentalizing it within ourselves and moving forward. Perhaps if I had joined the group earlier, the course of my emotional healing would not have been so drawn out. I certainly thought that could be the case for many. I was still very thankful for all of my time alone to come to terms with the physical, spiritual, and emotional conflicts within me. I could see how this could be very helpful for many cancer survivors in the early stages of treatment. It might even be beneficial to someone before they start treatment although at that time there were so many other things we needed to accomplish. I can certainly see the benefits of having one person to confide in who had been through the experience. That was something I yearned for when I was first diagnosed. I was isolated and felt sure that I was the only one in my position. This was so far from the truth. I would have liked to have had someone show me their mastectomy scars and show me their reconstructive surgical scars. I would like to have heard about chemotherapy and radiation from someone who had gone through it. Experience is a wonderful teacher whether someone else's or one's own.

Chapter 17

Contemplating Genetic Testing

While I was getting ready for the reunion and all my vacationing, I decided to pursue genetic counseling with a counselor and my oncologist. I was really interested in having the genetic testing done because my sister, my daughter, and my nieces were at a higher risk now for breast cancer and I felt as though I would like to do everything I could to put their minds at ease regarding the breast cancer. It was a difficult decision and I had some mixed emotions about giving my family too much information. The answer was not really black and white. I also did not want to negatively impact my ability to get health insurance.

After answering a very lengthy questionnaire and faxing it to another Rocky Mountain Cancer Center office, I set up an appointment with a genetics counselor. I spent a fair amount of time with her looking at all the data and trying to make an informed decision. I really did not think that I had a genetic predisposition to breast cancer and was prepared not to have the testing done but I did want to hear about the pros and cons.

Only about 10 percent of breast cancers are of the hereditary type. I did have a first cousin on my mother's side of the family who developed breast cancer at 34 years old, six months after the birth of her fifth child. That gave me one first degree relative that had developed breast cancer pre-menopausally. All of the other cancer history in my family seemed to be sporadic and unrelated, although we have had our fair share of cancer diagnoses. There was no other link to a possible genetic abnormality. With two women in my generation diagnosed with breast cancer at a young age(under age 50), the chance of a genetic mutation could be up to 80%, however the cause could be mutations other than the BRCA 1 or 2 that have yet to be discovered and studied.

Both BRCA-1 and BRCA-2 are autosomal dominant which means that only one of a chromosome pair needs to be affected to pass the susceptibility on to the next generation. The most engaging information I found was that women with BRCA-1 have a 60% chance of developing ovarian cancer and men an increased chance of prostate cancer. There was also a slightly increased incidence of cancer of the colon. BRCA-2 occurs somewhat less often and may only increase the chance of subsequent ovarian cancer by 20-25% and interestingly men with this also had an increased chance of breast cancer. The chance of these being inherited by the children of a parent positive for the gene is 50%.

It was my belief that knowing whether or not I was positive for either of these genes was only important if I planned to do something with the information. If I was not willing to share the results with the women in my family, then having the test done seemed unnecessary. I had not become any less proactive and I would certainly share the information with my family and I was prepared to have a prophylactic oophrectomy (removal of both ovaries) or even a total hysterectomy while they were in there to remove all risk of ovarian cancer. My ovaries right now caused me more trouble than they were worth because of the presence of some estrogen producing capability. Unfortunately estrogen is my enemy with estrogen receptor positive tumors. I made the difficult decisions and was prepared to have the blood drawn for the tests. The test was completed the week I got home from South Dakota and it would take a month to receive the results. I cannot overemphasize enough that genetic testing was not for everyone and my decision making process may not have been the best for other people but it worked for me. There were huge consequences with which I had to be prepared to deal when obtaining information of this magnitude.

My test results returned about four weeks after the blood was drawn and I tested negative for both genes. My risk for breast cancer existed because I was a woman and for no other reason. I felt a fair amount of relief and I did not even think I was even slightly anxious. My anxiety free lifestyle is certainly having good effects.

Regardless of the results of the tests, because of my breast cancer diagnosis, my female relatives moved into a high risk category which changed the guidelines for screening for breast cancer. They should begin mammography at age 25 or ten years before the youngest case of breast cancer in the family. They should have breast exams by a physician every six months starting at age 15 or 20. They should start monthly self-breast examinations at age 15. These are the recommendations of the Rocky Mountain Cancer Centers Genetic Counseling Service. I present them only as they affect my family. You can be sure I will teach my daughter as soon as she has breasts how to do a self -breast examination, not to frighten her but make her aware and give her confidence. My sister Janet was the one most at risk right now and I have encouraged her to be seen at a Cancer Center because there were several clinical trials going on with tamoxifen and other drugs given to female siblings of breast cancer patients as a preventive measure against developing breast cancer. She also chose to have testing for BRCA-1 and BRCA-2 and was found to be negative for both. She has been more reluctant to pursue a clinical trial for prevention.

Let me also point out that there were two very interesting research studies whose results have been released as I have been writing this book that show great promise. One involves the drug letrozole and its potential for decreasing recurrent cancer after the five years that patients require tamoxifen and another involves a vaccine for patients with late stage breast cancer that may have some effects when given earlier. I will be first in line when my five years on tamoxifen are over to take a similar drug with a promising outcome.

Chapter 18

One Year Anniversaries

As I approached my birthday and the year anniversaries of the events surrounding the diagnosis and treatment of my cancer, I had to pause and think about them. I remember so vividly that moment a year before when I found the first lump. I was a far different and much better person. One of the big milestones still ahead was the Race for the Cure. I was trying to train with a little running in addition to my regular workouts. I looked forward to what will surely be a very emotional day for me as I joined thousands of other breast cancer survivors. I hoped my family and Geri would have a really uplifting run or walk too. They've been there through it all and I wouldn't think of not having them at this race with me. Approaching the race as a milestone had made the journey interesting.

I had gone on my first long hike with my Rocky Mountain Team Survivor support group and it was wonderful. I was a little sore from hiking the hills but it was a beautiful hike through the foothills at the base of the Flatirons, which are beautiful mountainous rock formations overlooking Boulder. There were beautiful wildflowers even late in the summer. There was also evidence of bear activity. The group does a long hike once a month and last year went snow shoeing. I was going to have to prepare for another new experience.

I also found a Bible study that I thought might be a perfect match for me. Again I had prayed for something to help me in my daily devotional time and knew a little structure would definitely give me good direction. It took discipline for me to spend the necessary time studying but I was ready to take the time for Bible study. My faith had gotten me through the darkest hours in the past year.

As I approached my one year follow-up appointment with the oncologist, anxiety once gain overtook me, but only briefly. Blood would be drawn to make sure my liver wasn't a site of possible metastasis. I would also have a chest X-ray to check for lung metastasis. For the week or so before the appointment, I had a strange cough and I was a bit concerned about the chest x-ray. I was able to exercise and run and do all that my workout entailed so my activity was not restricted. I reasoned that it was normal that I would have a bit of anxiety. This made me nervous and I would be glad when the appointment was over, and I would hear the good word that everything was normal. I felt so good and so strong at that time. I still tired easily but even with my new less stressful view of life, it was a challenge for me to juggle all the balls of my life, deftly keeping them all in the air. As the appointment got closer my anxiety went up even with meditation and prayer. September 30th marked the one year anniversary of my first diagnosis of breast cancer. As I looked outside on a somewhat gloomy day, it was autumn and the leaves were turning and nothing could be more beautiful. I was so thankful to be here and have the last year behind me.

In getting ready for all of the milestones, my dad became very sick again. He had just returned from a trip and received an epidural injection for pain relief. As I hoped events were beginning to calm down, I arrived at his apartment to find him unresponsive. The nurses called an ambulance and he was transported to the Emergency Room where we spent the next six hours to find he had to have emergency surgery for a small bowel obstruction. I was concerned because his last surgery was a gut wrenching experience that marked the beginning of my fight against breast cancer. Although there may be no connection, I would always believe stress played a significant part in my health. My dad made it through surgery later to develop pneumonia from aspirating gastric contents, and then to end up with a second surgery to remove a necrotic and infected gall bladder. This led to a three week hospitalization and subsequent release to the nursing home for rehabilitation. My stress level elevated and my stomach churned with the agony of the year before. I prayed for peace but like a butterfly it was fleeting. My previous experiences were too fresh in my mind. I got confused as to whether it was this year or last. Now when I awakened from my dreams I was so thankful that it was still this year. I needed to cast my burdens on the Lord and leave them there. He would give me peace and answer my prayers. He has been there with me for the last year.

Apprehension and excitement preceded my appointment with the oncologist. My blood was drawn and my weight was checked just like every other visit. Awaiting the doctor looking around the exam room, I felt pretty calm. He came in and told me how great I looked and that my chest X-ray was normal. That was a huge relief. My cough just must be due to the dust around my house created by the workmen putting in the wood floors and the carpet being replaced. I never heard the results of my lab work, but assumed they were normal because no news was good news. I had been lulled into thinking that before but I believed it now. The doctor performed an exam and found nothing suspicious, but again he was very impressed with my breasts and I agreed that the outcome was amazing.

I really wanted to go work for my plastic surgeon. If I needed to go back to work I wanted to choose a very happy and relaxing situation. I also wanted to work with breast cancer patients. I was sure that acute care was not where I wanted to be, particularly since my dad had been in the hospital for weeks and had two surgeries and developed pneumonia. My head would have rolled if any post-operative patient of mine, ever in my career, developed pneumonia. Nurses now are overworked and understaffed. I would deal with the work situation later since my goal was to finish a book about my experiences and get it published before I forgot all the feelings and emotions. I also determined that I would be a breast cancer advocate in any way that I could. I vowed to make a difference.

My stress level had gone up significantly since my dad was hospitalized and I felt like I did last summer when I raced between hospital and nursing home and his apartment. My belief in the stress theory of illness would always concern me regarding my health. Perhaps the stress last summer that resulted in my cancer diagnosis was good since I found the lump and it most certainly did not just appear out of nowhere. It had surely been there for many years and maybe the stress just made it grow enough so I could feel it. That stress could have saved my life. I will never really know.

While my dad was in the hospital, I had a recurrence of my Benign Paroxysmal Positional Vertigo. I had been doing a lot of lifting and bending and moving heavy furniture which I suspected set it off as I was normally very careful to not do those things. I awakened in the middle of the night and got up to go to the bathroom and promptly fell right into the door. Then when I returned to bed I ran into the door jam. I made a fair amount of noise and Jim woke up to see what was wrong. He guessed what was going on immediately. This was not the first time we had been through this. I took some compazine (for the nausea) and carefully went back to bed and kept my head movement minimal. When I woke up in the morning I performed the maneuvers to get those particles to the area in the ear that did not cause the sensation of dizziness. The process was a bit excruciating since it caused severe nausea and usually vomiting. The relief was almost instantaneous and although I felt a little spacey for a day, I knew I would ultimately feel better. The most difficulty encountered was sleeping sitting up at a 45 degree angle, for 48 hours, but I usually managed that. Luckily the BPPV predated my breast cancer or I would be absolutely sure I had brain metastasis. Because of my nursing background, I knew there were no simple diagnoses. I just hoped I was walking on level ground before the Race for the Cure. Even if I had to crawl, I would participate.

What I knew was that I needed to decrease my stress and get some order back in my life once again. My dad finally was discharged to the nursing home after three weeks in the hospital. My sister and brother had both been to visit but the brunt of my dad's care rested on my shoulders. I hired an aide to be with him eighteen to twenty four hours a day and they would follow him to the nursing home. This gave me some peace of mind since I did not want him to fall. Amazingly while he was in the hospital, he fell and somehow the nurses made me feel responsible so the aides were hired sooner than later. He was not hurt, thank goodness. Unfortunately Harv and Janet actually had to go home and I had to adjust to life as the sole caretaker, once again. At least I had the nursing home and my aides to help take care of him. He ended up falling three more times before I got someone with him 24 hours a day. Somehow it was so hard to believe that no one could help him when his call light went on. Unless I actually walked a mile in their shoes I should not cast dispersions on the situation. My dad tended to be very impatient and impetuous.

Chapter 19

Race for the Cure

The Race for the Cure was only a day away and I was filled with anticipation and excitement. I had looked forward to this day for over a year. We had a great dinner with three kinds of fish; tuna, mahi mahi, and walleye. We did not really carbohydrate load since the race was only 3.1 miles. Geri cooked the meal for us. Although we were all anxious for tomorrow, we tried to get to bed early since we had to get up at 5:30 am. I signed up for the 7:30 am race, which was the survivor's race and the rest of the family started at 8:45 am. I had a great deal of difficulty sleeping and I eventually took a sleeping pill so that I could sleep. I felt like this was such a big day for me. It was the culmination of a year of trials and I hoped the beginning of the rest of my long life.

We left the house at 6:15 am seemingly with plenty of time, however the traffic was bumper to bumper and barely crept along. I jumped out of the car and ran to the beginning of the race. I was not really late but I wanted to pick up my pink survivor hat and my pink survivor T-shirt. I would not run this race without the pink hat. I put it on as soon as I got it and never took it off. I got to the beginning of the race and found my running time with the 9-10 minute milers.

I was all by myself and that was the way I wanted it. It's how it had to be. No matter how many people were around me, this was a journey I would take alone. My group of family and friends had been wonderfully supportive, but ultimately I had to get through this with only God watching over me. My emotions were so mixed. The journey of the last year had filled me with hope, love, and fear.

I felt a little anxious. I thought I would be really relieved at a year out and I found that I was not as calm as I would have liked to be. That made me anxious too. Did I choose the best chemotherapy? Should I have received more chemotherapy? I received the gold standard of treatment but I guess one is never totally comfortable when it was supposed to be all over. Also, when I stopped seeing the oncologist as frequently it was a bit unnerving. There was a great deal of comfort knowing you would see the doctor every few weeks or months. I still only had a ten year survival rate of 68.9%, according to the Mayo Clinic website. That was just not very reassuring, but then again the odds were in my favor. I did not like the odds anyway. I wanted to bet on me, not statistics, and I was strong and believed I would survive. Luckily I did not dwell on statistics but on finding life after resolving death.

The horn blew signaling the beginning of the race. It took me several minutes just to reach the starting line. Everywhere I looked there was a sea of pink. There were thousands of people. Some were running and some were walking. I went by young women who were pushing strollers who have on survivor hats. Wow, some of these women were too young to have had to deal with breast cancer. I felt pretty good in the early part of the run since I had not started out too quickly. I was not winded from the beginning as I had been in some races so I paced myself from the beginning. As I looked around, I was amazed by the number of people with the *In celebration of* and *In memory of* placards on their backs. So many people had died from this disease. So many people had survived this disease as well. So many people had been touched by this disease.

I never knew if we should call ourselves survivors. Perhaps that is a bit presumptuous. We never really know if we still have the disease somewhere in our bodies waiting for a chance to appear. Maybe there is something else we should be calling ourselves. But for now, I felt like a survivor and the excitement of those around me gave me the energy to continue in the race. It is only when we get to ten years cancer free that we are considered cured and that was still a long time away for me. Even that was arbitrary since a recurrence could happen anywhere at anytime. I had trouble calling myself a survivor but I survived a lot from tragedy to triumph. There were no accurate markers to evaluate, to ensure that I would not have a recurrence. I thought I could only consider myself in remission but that was not a term I had heard relative to breast cancer, at least not recently. I knew they used that term in the leukemias. I was not really sure what to call myself except brave and enduring and patient. I had endured the diagnosis and the surgery and the rehabilitation. I had survived my High School reunion and letting all in attendance know of my trials, which was not an easy undertaking. I had everything going for me when I was in High School and like all young people thought I was invincible. Suddenly I was forced to deal with the harshest reality. I had survived multiple surgeries to complete my breast reconstruction which had been difficult at best, but rewarding as I looked at the final result. It's not really a conclusion because the scars kept forming and I might need more surgery, in fact probably would, to release the scar formation. I had not figured out what I wanted to do with the rest of my life but I felt like a little kid in a candy store right now, because I had so many choices. My mind was rapidly reviewing the last year as I continued the race.

I started to get a little tired at about two miles, but there were many people along the route that kept cheering everyone along, so that no matter how tired I felt I would not stop running. As I came around the final curve I could see the finish line and there was a river of pink between me and the finish line. Now it was just sheer determination that kept me going and I started to cry as I ran. Luckily I was so sweaty no one noticed. These were tears of absolute joy. Now the sounds of the crowd were deafening, but I heard my name. I looked up and saw my neighbor, Linda, and her daughter, Jill, as they shouted words of encouragement to me and then I saw Jim and Kate with balloons everywhere cheering me on. What a thrill! I was finally finished and as I slowed to a walk a little girl handed me a pink carnation and congratulated me. Running this race was like living the last year over again with the same victorious outcome. My time was about 45 minutes and I was quite happy with that. We could not delay at the end because the rest of the group was going to start their race in a few minutes. I walked them all over to the starting line and we picked up my friend Nancy and her son Dylan along the way. They had come to do this with me and for me. As always the kids took off quickly with Jim and Nancy right on their heels so Geri was left to walk alone, so I decided that I would walk the course again with her. This time I could relax and talk and laugh along the way. My journey was finished or maybe it was just beginning. This time as I approached the finish line doves were released in memory of all those who had died from this disease. They were a beautiful white against the bright blue Colorado sky. As they flew toward heaven I felt the presence of all of the women with breast cancer, both those living and those who had died. I was so moved that I was speechless.

Chapter 20

The End of the Beginning

The impact of this past year on my life was extraordinary. My spiritual life had changed most. I had always considered myself a Christian and was born again years ago but I kept learning that God had the only true answers and if we were not open to them we missed them altogether. I had learned to count answers to my prayers rather than the prayers, and I had learned that in all things we must be very patient. I am not sure why I had breast cancer but I knew there was a reason. I knew that my experiences had already taught people that they too could survive this diagnosis if they or a loved one were to get it. When I was first diagnosed I was scared to death of chemotherapy and now I knew that I could survive that as well. It might not have been pleasant but the cancer did not win, I did. My spirit was eternal. The experience may well prove to be my defining moment. I was a better Christian woman as a result of my diagnosis.

My life was better for having had breast cancer. Well, maybe not better, but I had certainly learned many valuable lessons. Having found the lump early probably saved my life. I lived each day to the fullest and took nothing for granted. Our health was as much a gift as life itself. God had not forsaken me but blessed me abundantly. I had endured much but gained more. I hoped that I had tremendous insight into the lives of those around me. Life was fleeting but eternity, unending. I did not want to go there quite yet but I had learned to die. Not in a morbid sense but in a very heavenly sense. I had to learn to die before I could resolve to learn to live again and live was what I chose to do for as long as the good Lord gave me on this earth.

I continued to pray for my children and my husband and my family and for the times I was here as well as for the times I might not be here. I had been forced to prepare my family at least on paper for the time when I might not be with them and planned for their lives and continued strength as well as for their financial future and their future without me. I did not want them to forget me, but I did not want them to be paralyzed by grief. I made sure that while I was undergoing chemotherapy that I was completing their scrapbooks and giving them a family legacy on which they could build. I cannot imagine anything worse than leaving nothing to my children. I wanted and needed to leave a legacy and God had answered my prayers and helped me to do that by finishing the scrapbooks to the present and by getting my proverbial house in order. I needed to do that literally, too. I felt a great need to put my house in order.

The obvious was getting new wood floors, carpet and furniture. The not so obvious was teaching my children to pray for answers and expect those answers. I wanted them to see what God had done in my life. I wanted to be here for many years to come but the only way for me to do that was to prepare to leave right away and in that regard I hoped I could relax and enjoy every minute, hour and day, no matter how many there would be. Being prepared for the unexpected was something we should all accomplish. I credited being in the military for having given my husband and I both a reason to complete a will, decide a custodian for our children, and prepare for everyone's financial future. As part of the preparation for deployment each military member must have all of these things prepared. It was very matter of fact and did not become a tortured task since we generally prepared it far before the need for it might arise.

Emotionally, I had been through every conceivable emotion in the past year. Having been through the loss of a parent, loss of a friend and physician, loss of body parts, loss of hair, loss of my blissful ignorance and naivety, and a potential loss of my own life had been overwhelming. I had been on the brink of terror, awakened in a panic, in the depths of depression, and frightened beyond comprehension. My anger had been paralyzing and my grief immeasurable. I felt as though the better part of a year was spent in tears with fears of going out, staying in, getting sick, being seen in public, not being seen in public, facing cancer, facing my friends, and being that *poor* woman with breast cancer. I had also experienced extraordinary joy at having a wonderfully supportive family and friends and feeling the immense sense of accomplishment at having completed an enormous task. I was proud to have been productive and proactive.

I had a rewarding profession that had given me an opportunity to speak to women in informal groups and settings and one-on-one to educate them about all of the aspects of breast cancer and to teach them to be vigilant with their own health and use all of the early assessment tools we have to catch this curable disease early. I had been honored to have the privilege of making new friends who have suffered this type of cancer and other types as well. As the group leader of Rocky Mountain Team Survivor-Boulder, Dora Briegleb says, "It is a pretty good sorority to join. However, you must go through some horrible initiation rights." I have been touched by the bravery and resolve of other cancer victims to never give up, their candor during support group meetings, as well as their immediate love and acceptance of newcomers was a true blessing.

Physically, I had gone from peak fitness to barely being able to get out of bed. I had a major surgical procedure that I was not sure I even wanted. I had struggled to start to regain my activity level only to be beaten down by each chemotherapy treatment and to have to start all over again. I'd had muscles tighten so much that my posture was affected. I have been so uncomfortable that I was sure nothing would ever function correctly again. I endured uncomfortable physical therapy to try to loosen muscles and regain good posture. I had gone through menopause and not lost my mind or my sense of humor.

I had become a part of the health care system in a role I never wanted and definitely did not choose. That role was being a cancer patient. I had gone through countless hours of research and put together the best medical and surgical team available. I had been faced with medical decisions with life threatening consequences. I had felt the guilt of not going into a clinical research study. I was a nurse, and education and research should be a top priority for me. I had reached the end of traditional therapy and wondered if that was all there was? I had asked the question of myself, "Did I do enough?" Maybe I should have had more chemotherapy and maybe radiation. I had seen the devastation that a diagnosis of cancer could have on finances. I had experienced the health insurance conundrum. I had been appalled at the cost of medical care and disgusted by the value society and the insurance companies placed on that care. I had seen generous charities help cancer patients pay for much needed life saving chemotherapy and a few that would also pay for not so necessary treatments that just made you feel better.

I cannot think of a better way to end this book except by telling the story of my daughter going to school the day after the Race for the Cure. She had gotten a hockey puck at the race and was taking it to school for show and tell. She proudly wore her Race for the Cure shirt and told the class that she had run the race the day before and had received the hockey puck for finishing.

Then she announced to the class, "My mother is a survivor."

Author's note

As I went through this experience I began to pray that God would direct me down a path. The path He wanted me to be on. I wanted Him to show me what it was that I needed to do to leave a legacy in this world. I prayed that everyday and one of the answers I received was the reason for this book. This is my testimony to Him. I wanted to be a witness to God's love and I never knew how I personally could do that. I did not do well carrying around my soapbox. I was not a charismatic speaker just a truthful one. I wanted my children to see me each day living what I taught and believed. I wanted them to see me pray and reach out to God for answers and help in good times and bad. I wanted them to see me thank and praise Him for all the blessings and answered prayers that I saw everyday. I also wanted to be a blessing to other people who may be going through an experience just like mine. Through this book I would like my faith to shine for all to see. I have survived through God's love.

A few scripture passages have given me tremendous strength. From Matthew 7: 7-8, "Ask, and it shall be given to you; seek, and you shall find; knock, and it shall be opened to you. For everyone who asks receives, and he who seeks finds, and to him who knocks it shall be opened." From Philippians 4: 6-7, "Be anxious for nothing but in everything by prayer and supplication with thanksgiving let your requests be made known to God. And the peace of God which surpasses all comprehension shall guard your hearts and your minds through Christ Jesus." And from Isaiah 40: 31, "Yet those who wait for the Lord will gain new strength; they will mount up with wings like eagles, they will run and not get tired, they will walk and not become weary."

I hope as I carry the message of early detection of breast cancer and survival with God, I can leave a legacy to my children and anyone who reads this book.

I am now a four year survivor. I have had a few scares along the way, but am cancer free, at least today. I have gone back to work with my very understanding Plastic Surgeon, Dr Debora Ma, and my greatest joy is working with our cancer patients, especially those with breast cancer who I hope benefit from the wisdom of my experience.